BODY FLUIDS

Laboratory Examination of Cerebrospinal,
Synovial, and Serous Fluids: A Textbook Atlas

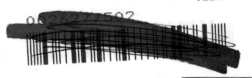

TELEPEN

BODY FLUIDS

Laboratory Examination of Cerebrospinal,
Synovial, and Serous Fluids: A Textbook Atlas

Carl R. Kjeldsberg, MD

Professor of pathology and
chief of hematopathology
Department of Pathology
University of Utah College
of Medicine, Salt Lake City

Joseph A. Knight, MD

Associate professor of pathology
and director of clinical pathology
Department of Pathology
University of Utah College
of Medicine, Salt Lake City

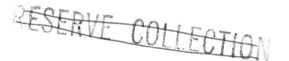
Educational Products Division
American Society of Clinical Pathologists
Chicago

ASCP
AMERICAN SOCIETY OF CLINICAL PATHOLOGISTS INC.
1922

Notice

Trade names for equipment and supplies described herein are included as suggestions only. In no way does their inclusion constitute an endorsement or preference by the American Society of Clinical Pathologists. The ASCP did not test the equipment, supplies, or procedures and, therefore, urges all readers to read and follow all manufacturers' instructions and package insert warnings concerning the proper and safe use of products.

Library of Congress Cataloging in Publication Data

Kjeldsberg, Carl R.
  Body fluids.

  Includes bibliographical references and index.
    1. Body fluids—Analysis.   2. Body fluids—Examination.   3. Body fluids—Examination—Atlases.   I. Knight, Joseph A., 1930-   . II. Title. [DNLM: 1. Body fluids—Analysis—Atlases.   QY 17 K62b]
  RB52.K56   616.07′56   81-14837
  ISBN 0-89189-104-8   AACR2

To our wives, Gillean and Pauline

Contents

Preface

Until now, the information on body fluids has been sparse and fragmented. Anyone seeking a thorough understanding of the subject had to consult multiple references to tap all the laboratory resources available for thoroughly examining fluid specimens.

While serum and urine have received adequate coverage in medical literature, other fluids have not fared as well. That is why we have concentrated on the laboratory investigation of cerebrospinal, synovial, and serous fluids—to fill the need for a comprehensive text that explains the basic principles and methods of examining these fluids in a concise, yet thorough, manner.

This book is based on a manual that we prepared a few years ago for a workshop on body fluids. It has been expanded and updated to serve as a relevant reference for pathologists, pathology residents, and medical technologists. While it is intended for clinical laboratories, it could also be useful in workshop and classroom settings.

The purpose of the book is to provide a narrative and pictorial description of cell morphology; methodology on how to collect, store, and examine specimens; and guidelines for selecting various tests according to their diagnostic significance. The photomicrographs depict smears prepared by the cytocentrifuge method and treated with Wright's (Romanovsky's) stain.

We are especially grateful to the following: Joe Marty, MS, MT (ASCP) for the microphotography; Britt Adams, MT (ASCP) and Mr. Marty for assistance in writing the methodology section; and Gwenevere South for typing the manuscript.

Carl R. Kjeldsberg, MD
Joseph A. Knight, MD

1 Cerebrospinal Fluid

Anatomy and Physiology

The brain and spinal cord are covered by three meningeal membranes, which are as follows from the outside inward: dura mater, arachnoid mater, and pia mater. Cerebrospinal fluid (CSF) is present in the subarachnoid space between the arachnoid mater and the pia mater and circulates over the cerebral hemispheres and downward over the spinal cord. Most of the CSF is formed by the choroid plexuses through ultrafiltration and active secretion. Extrachoroidal sites such as the ependymal lining of the ventricles and the cerebral subarachnoid space are other sources of CSF formation. Absorption of the CSF occurs through the arachnoid villi.

The total CSF volumes are 90–150 ml in adults and 10–60 ml in neonates. There is a constant turnover of CSF with 50–500 ml being formed every 24 hours.[1]

The CSF acts as a protective cushion for the underlying central nervous tissue. Other functions of the CSF include collection of wastes, circulation of nutrients, and lubrication of the CNS.

The choroid plexus epithelium and the endothelium of capillaries in contact with CSF represent the anatomic aspect of the blood-CSF barrier. The endothelium of capillaries regulates the passage of various substances into the CSF from the blood. Reference values for the normal components of CSF are presented in Table 1–1.

Lumbar Puncture

Most studies on the CSF are based on a lumbar puncture, which is a relatively simple procedure. However, since potential complications may occur, the procedure should only be done for specific diagnostic or therapeutic purposes (Table 1–2). Prior to the spinal puncture, a careful clinical history and physical examination should be done. Particular attention should be paid to the examination of the optic fundi for evidence of increased intracranial pressure. If increased pressure is present, great care must be taken when removing fluid since herniation of the uncus through the tentorium cerebelli or the cerebellar tonsils through the foramen magnum may occur. When a spinal puncture is performed in the presence of increased intracranial pressure, neurosurgical consultation should be available.

A spinal puncture is contraindicated if there is infection at the proposed puncture site, as this may result in the spread of the infection into the meninges. Septicemia or a general systemic infection is a relative contraindication because spinal puncture may result in meningitis.

After the puncture is performed and before any fluid is withdrawn, a manometer is attached to record the opening pressure of the CSF. The normal pressure is

Table 1–1. Normal Reference Values for Cerebrospinal Fluid*†

Components‡	Conventional Units	SI Units
Albumin	10–30 mg/dl	100–300 mg/liter
Calcium	2.1–2.7 mEq/liter	1.05–1.35 mmole/liter
Chloride	115–130 mEq/liter	115–130 mmole/liter
Glucose	50–80 mg/dl	2.75–4.40 mmole/liter
Lactate	10–25 mg/dl	1.11–2.81 mmole/liter
Leukocyte count	0–5 mononuclear cells/μl	0–0.005 × 10^9/liter
Leukocyte differential		
Adults		
Lymphocytes	60% ± 20	
Monocytes	30% ± 15	
Neutrophils	2% ± 4	
Neonates		
Lymphocytes	20% ± 15	
Monocytes	70% ± 20	
Neutrophils	4% ± 4	
Total protein	15–45 mg/dl	150–450 mg/liter

*Data adapted from Krieg.[2] Used by permission.
†Except where noted for the leukocyte differential, reference values apply to adults.
‡Reliable values for enzymes have not yet been established. Lactic dehydrogenase has been reported to be approximately 10% of serum levels.

Table 1–2. Indications for Lumbar Puncture

Suspected Conditions
Meningitis, encephalitis, syphilis, brain abscess
Subarachnoid and intracerebral hemorrhage
Multiple sclerosis, Guillain-Barré syndrome
Acute leukemia and lymphoma with CNS involvement
Spinal cord and brain tumor

Therapy
Chemotherapy for leukemia and lymphoma
Introduction of anesthetics, radiographic-contrast media
Amphotericin therapy in fungal meningitis

Table 1–3. Causes of Cerebrospinal Fluid Pressure Changes

Increased
Congestive heart failure
Meningitis
Thrombosis of venous sinuses
Superior vena cava obstruction
Cerebral edema
Mass lesion (abscess, tumor, cerebral hemorrhage)
Hypo-osmolality
Impairment of CSF absorption

Decreased
Spinal-subarachnoid block
Dehydration
Circulatory collapse
CSF leakage

50–180 mm when the patient is in a lateral position but slightly higher in a sitting position. Small transient changes in the pressure are noted with respiration, coughing, and straining. These changes are normal and indicate patency of the channels through which the CSF flows. The CSF pressure may be decreased or increased in a variety of disorders[1] (Table 1–3). If the pressure is normal, up to 20 ml can be removed without danger. Ideally, the specimen should be divided into three samples placed in sterile tubes, which are labeled sequentially. Tube 1 should be used for chemical and immunologic studies, tube 2 for microbiologic examination, and tube 3 for a cell count. If the initial pressure is greater than 200 mm, not more than 2 ml of CSF

should be removed. Before removing the spinal puncture needle, the closing pressure should be recorded.

Gross Examination

The CSF is normally clear and colorless. If a disease is present, the fluid may have a cloudy, turbid, or bloody appearance. Cloudy or turbid fluid may be due to pleocytosis (leukocyte count > 200/μl), microorganisms, RBCs (> 400 cells/μl), or increased protein.

Following injection of radiographic-contrast medium, the CSF may have an oily appearance. A fat embolism in the brain may be associated with fat globules of varying sizes in the CSF.

When the CSF is pinkish red, this usually indicates the presence of blood, which may have resulted from subarachnoid hemorrhage, intracerebral hemorrhage, infarct, or traumatic tap. It is, of course, extremely important to differentiate traumatic tap from pathologic bleeding. The following observations are useful in differentiating these two mechanisms from one another: (1) A traumatic tap shows maximum blood in the first sample with a progressive decrease in subsequent samples. Generally, in subarachnoid hemorrhage, the blood is evenly mixed in the three tubes. The presence of crenated RBCs is not useful in differentiating traumatic tap from pathologic bleeding. (2) After the CSF is centrifuged, the supernatant fluid is clear in a traumatic tap, but it is xanthochromic in a subarachnoid hemorrhage. (3) A clot may be seen in the CSF when there is a very bloody traumatic tap, while subarachnoid hemorrhage per se is usually not associated with clot formation. It should be noted, however, that traumatic and subarachnoid bleeding may be concurrent, and that the supernatant fluid may be clear for the first three hours after the onset of subarachnoid hemorrhage. In addition, a markedly traumatic tap may be associated with some blood and xanthochromia of the CSF two to five days following the initial puncture.

Xanthochromia of the CSF refers to a pink, orange, or yellow color of the supernatant after the CSF has been centrifuged. Two to four hours after a subarachnoid hemorrhage, lysis of the RBCs occurs. This gives a pale orange color to the supernatant due to the release of oxyhemoglobin. Within 24 hours, hemoglobin is converted to bilirubin, giving a yellowish tint to the supernatant. Bilirhachia usually reaches a peak in about 36 hours and may persist for several weeks. In addition to subarachnoid hemorrhage, there are other causes of xanthochromia, as shown in Table 1–4.[2]

Table 1–4. Causes of Xanthochromia

Subarachnoid and intracerebral hemorrhage
Traumatic tap
Jaundice
Elevated protein (>150 mg/dl)
Premature birth
Hypercarotenemia
Meningeal melanoma

Normal CSF does not clot; however, clotting may be seen when the CSF protein content is sharply elevated as with Froin's syndrome and with a very bloody traumatic tap.

Cell Counts

The cell counts are performed in a counting chamber with undiluted CSF. Electronic cell counters should not be used for the CSF since there is poor precision in the normal range. The normal leukocyte counts are 0–5 mononuclear leukocytes/μl in adults, 0–30/μl in children less than 1 year of age, 0–20/μl in children 1 to 4 years of age, and 0–10/μl in children 5 years of age to puberty.[2,3] It should be pointed out, however, that there is no general agreement on the normal values for children.[4] For obvious reasons, it is difficult to arrive at a reliable set of normal CSF leukocyte values.

If a traumatic tap is suspected, RBC counts on the CSF may be used to correct CSF leukocyte counts or CSF protein determinations. This correction, however, is valid only if the cell count and the total protein concentration are determined in the same tube of CSF.[2] In addition, it should be noted that this correction is an approximation and limited by the precision of the CSF red blood cell count. The following formula may be used:

$$W = WBC_f - \frac{WBC_b \times RBC_f}{RBC_b}$$

where:

W = CSF leukocyte count before the blood was added
WBC_f = total CSF leukocyte count
RBC_f = total CSF red blood cell count
RBC_b = red blood cell count in the blood
WBC_b = leukocyte count in the blood

In general, with a normal peripheral blood count, this correction amounts to approximately 1–2 leukocytes/1,000 RBCs.[2]

Similarly, a calculation of the true CSF protein content can be made in a traumatic tap by using a correction factor of 1 mg/dl for every 1,200 RBCs/μl.[2] This is assuming, however, that the patient has a normal hematocrit and normal serum protein.

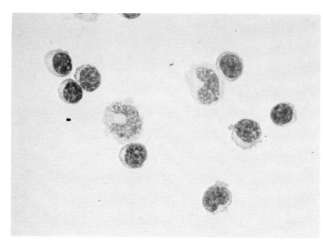

Fig 1. Two monocytes and several lymphocytes.

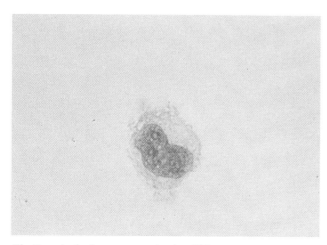

Fig 2. A single monocyte in the CSF.

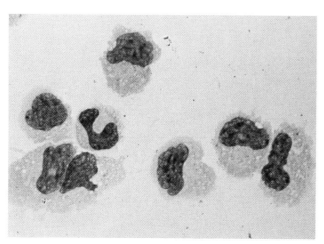

Fig 3. Several monocytes in the CSF.

Differential Count

A differential count should be done on a stained smear made from the CSF. A "chamber differential" is unsatisfactory as one cannot be certain of the cell types present in a wet preparation. Furthermore, concentration of the CSF on a smear provides a larger number of cells, and proper staining will allow an accurate identification of the cell types present. Normal values are quoted in Table 1–5.

Table 1–5.   Normal Cerebrospinal Fluid Differential Count*

Cell Type	Adults	Neonates
Lymphocytes	60% ± 20	20% ± 15
Monocytes	30% ± 15	70% ± 20
Neutrophils	2% ± 4	4% ± 4†
Neuroectodermal cells	rare	rare

*Sedimentation or cytocentrifuge methods used. Data adapted from Krieg[2] and Sheth.[5]
†In high-risk neonates without meningitis, the CSF may have ± 60% neutrophils. Data from Sarff, Platt, and McCracken.[3]

Recently, many new techniques have been introduced that increase the cellular yield and provide satisfactory morphology. These include filter techniques, sedimentation methods, and cytocentrifugation. (These methods are discussed in the Appendix.)

It is recommended that stained smears be made on all CSF specimens even though the total cell count is within normal limits. Using 0.5 ml of normal CSF, approximately 30–50 cells are usually obtained by the cytocentrifuge or sedimentation method.[5, 6]

Normal Cells

A few *RBCs* are frequently found in the CSF due to contamination by blood from vessels injured during the lumbar puncture. The CSF normally contains a small number of *lymphocytes* and *monocytes* (Figs 1 through 3). There is some disagreement in the literature regarding the ratio of lymphocytes to monocytes. This probably is due to the different methods used in preparing the smears. Recent literature cites the ratio of lymphocytes to monocytes as being approximately 70:30.[7] In young children the CSF has a higher percentage of monocytes, and up to 80% may be normal. Reticulomonocytes, meningeal histiocytoid cells, and pia-arachnoid mesothelial cells are other terms used for monocytes in CSF. The origin of lymphocytes and monocytes in CSF is uncertain. Some authors believe that they originate from leptomeningeal stem cells, while others suspect that they originate from the blood.[7]

There is also disagreement as to whether *polymorphonuclear leukocytes (PMNs)* occur in normal CSF. The older literature indicates that any PMNs in the CSF are indicative of disease. However, since the introduction of new techniques for concentrating the CSF, there have been reports that a small number of PMNs may be present in normal CSF.[5] Our experience confirms this. Using the cytocentrifuge, up to 10% neutrophils has been quoted as being normal.[5] The same investigator believes that the presence of PMNs is clinically significant only if the total leukocyte count exceeds 10 cells/μl. It is also possible that the neutrophils in CSF come from contamination by peripheral blood through a traumatic tap. In general, it is recommended that one should relate the presence of a small number of PMNs to the clinical situation and the results of other laboratory tests.[2]

Ependymal cells from the ventricular lining and *choroidal plexus* cells may occasionally be seen in normal and abnormal CSF. From a cytologic viewpoint, it is difficult to differentiate ependymal from choroidal plexus cells.[7] Both are usually seen in clusters and are uniform in size, shape, and appearance. The nuclei are the size of a small lymphocyte; while the cytoplasm is abundant, cloudy, and gray-blue. The nuclear chromatin is delicate (Figs 4 and 5). It is important to be able to recognize these cells because they may be mistaken for malignant cells. The ependymal and choroidal plexus cells are more frequently seen in CSF obtained by cisternal or ventricular puncture than by a lumbar puncture. They may be seen following trauma, surgery, pneumoencephalography, myelography, or ischemic infarction of the brain. Their presence is of little diagnostic value.[7, 8]

Additional cell types that may be found in the normal CSF include *cartilage cells* and *bone marrow cells* (Fig 6).[8] The presence of such cells has no diagnostic significance and is caused by accidental puncture of the vertebral body. In rare cases, *squamous epithelial cells* from the skin may also be observed.

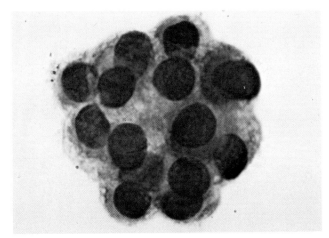

Fig 4. A cluster of choroid plexus cells.

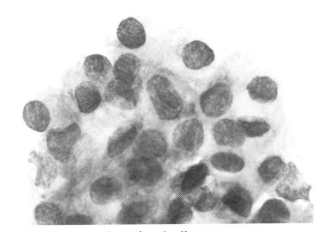

Fig 5. A cluster of ependymal cells.

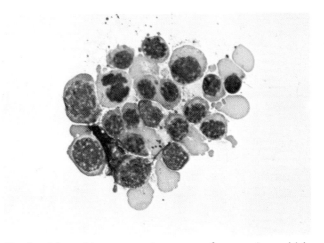

Fig 6. Normoblasts at varying stages of maturation, which are present in the CSF due to accidental puncture of the vertebral body.

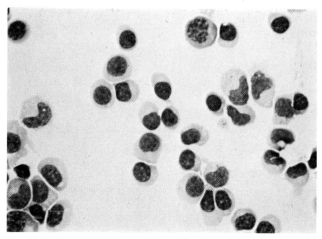

Fig 7. Lymphocytosis of the CSF and a few monocytes in a patient with viral meningitis.

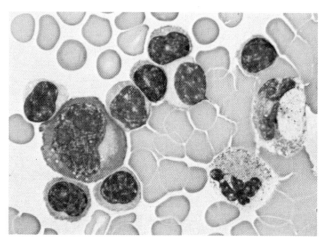

Fig 8. Lymphocytes, granulocytes, and a large mononuclear cell from a patient recovering from viral meningitis. The large mononuclear cell is a reactive or transformed lymphocyte (immunoblast).

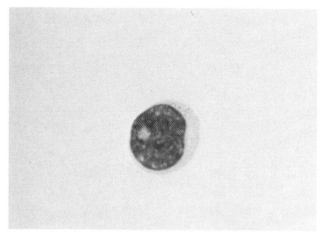

Fig 9. A lymphoblast in the CSF of a newborn.

Abnormal Cells

Lymphocytes in the CSF have a similar appearance to their counterparts in the blood and transform in a similar fashion when confronted by an antigen. Thus, a spectrum of lymphoid cells may be seen, including lymphocytes of varying sizes (Fig 7), plasmacytoid lymphocytes, plasma cells, immunoblasts, and lymphoblasts.[7, 8] It may be difficult to identify lymphocytes when marked reactive changes are present. The stimulated, reactive, or transformed lymphocyte is large and has basophilic cytoplasm and moderately coarse chromatin with one or more nucleoli (Fig 8). The immature appearing lymphocyte or lymphoblast has scant cytoplasm, a delicate chromatin pattern, and nucleoli that may or may not be prominent. Atypical, reactive, or transformed lymphocytes are commonly seen in patients with viral meningitis. Lymphoblasts may be noted in CSF from newborns and neonates (Fig 9). The most helpful feature in differentiating benign lymphoid cells from malignant cells is that there is usually a mixture of small, large, and transformed lymphocytes in benign cases; while malignant cells are more uniform. Lymphocytosis of the CSF is seen in a variety of infectious and noninfectious diseases (Table 1–6).[2] Cell surface marker studies have shown that the lymphocyte subpopulations (B and T cells) in the CSF parallel those seen in the peripheral blood. In inflammatory diseases the CSF lymphocytes are primarily T-lymphocytes.[9–11]

Table 1–6.   Causes of Cerebrospinal Fluid Lymphocytic Pleocytosis*

Viral meningoencephalitis
Aseptic meningitis
Tuberculous meningoencephalitis (mixed-cell reaction)
Partially treated bacterial meningitis
Syphilitic meningoencephalitis
Leptospiral meningitis (often mixed reaction)
Fungal meningitis (mixed-cell reaction)
Parasitic disease
Multiple sclerosis
Guillain-Barré syndrome
Polyneuritis
Sarcoidosis of meninges
*Data adapted from Krieg.[2] Used by permission.

Plasma cells are not seen in normal CSF and their presence suggests an inflammatory process (Fig 10). They are especially seen in acute viral diseases and certain chronic inflammatory conditions such as tuberculosis, syphilis, sarcoidosis, subacute sclerosing panencephalitis, and multiple sclerosis.[7, 8]

Monocytes are usually present in increased numbers together with neutrophils and lymphocytes. Such a mixed reaction is seen in a variety of disorders (Table 1–7).[2, 8] A pure monocytosis in the CSF is rarely seen.

Table 1–7.   Causes of Cerebrospinal Fluid Monocytic Pleocytosis*†

Chronic bacterial meningitis
Partially treated bacterial meningitis
Syphilitic meningoencephalitis
Viral meningoencephalitis
Fungal meningitis
Leptospiral meningitis
Amebic encephalomyelitis
CNS hemorrhage
Cerebral infarct
Multiple sclerosis
Reaction to foreign material
CNS malignancies
*Data adapted from Krieg.[2] Used by permission.
†Usually associated with mixed-cell reactions.

Macrophages in CSF are thought to develop from pluripotential stem cells in the reticuloendothelial tissue of the leptomeninges and from monocytes.[7] Macrophages may be seen to phagocytose red cells, leukocytes, other macrophages, microorganisms, pigments, and lipids.[8] The material that has been phagocytosed is acted upon by enzymes. That which cannot be utilized by the macrophage is often stored in the cytoplasm in the form of vacuoles. These vacuoles may fuse and push the nucleus to the periphery, forming a so-called signet ring. Such cells may measure up to 100 μ in diameter.[8]

Hemorrhage is associated with the appearance of neutrophils and many macrophages; the latter phagocytose RBCs within a few hours (Figs 11 and 12). The phagocytosed red cells rapidly lose their color and appear as empty vacuoles in the cytoplasm of the macrophages (Fig 13). After approximately four days, hemosiderin is seen as dark brown or black granules (Fig 14).[7, 8] Later, hematoidin pigment may be seen as brownish yellow or sometimes red crystals (Fig 15). Iron within a macrophage *(siderophage)* may be demonstrated with an iron stain (Fig 16). The presence of several such siderophages is usually a good indication that hemorrhage has occurred.[8] Siderophages may still be

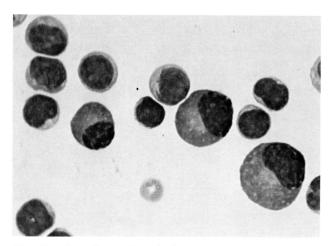

Fig 10.   Lymphocytosis and plasmacytosis in a patient with multiple sclerosis.

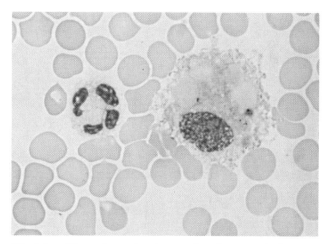

Fig 11.   Macrophage showing erythrophagocytosis in a patient with subarachnoid hemorrhage.

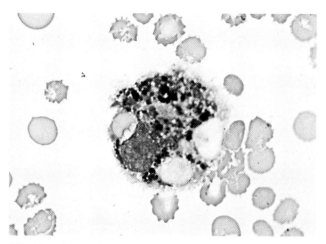

Fig 12.   Macrophage with phagocytosed RBCs and hemosiderin pigment from a patient with recurrent subarachnoid hemorrhage.

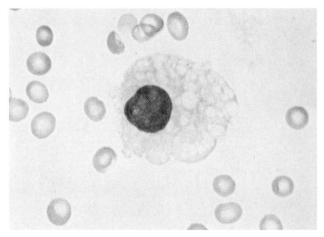

Fig 13. Macrophage with multiple phagocytic vacuoles.

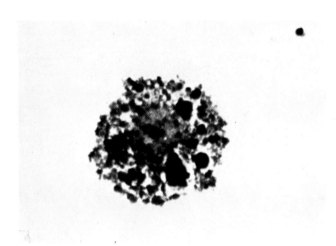

Fig 14. Macrophage (siderophage) containing multiple black granules, some of them representing hemosiderin, in a patient with subarachnoid hemorrhage.

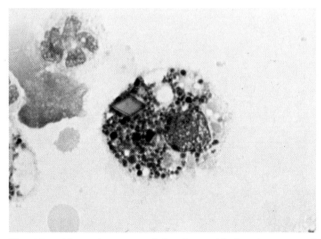

Fig 15. Macrophage containing hemosiderin pigment and a yellow hematoidin crystal from a patient with subarachnoid hemorrhage.

present several months after hemorrhage occurred.[8] The presence of a single macrophage showing erythrophagocytosis is not an absolute indicator of hemorrhage. Erythrophagocytosis may also occur in vitro or may be due to blood contamination of the CSF from a puncture repeated 8–12 hours following the initial lumbar puncture.[8] However, large numbers of macrophages showing erythrophagocytosis and several siderophages are good evidence that pathologic hemorrhage has occurred. Furthermore, the presence of erythrophagocytosis and siderophages in the CSF a week or longer following the initial hemorrhage is highly suggestive of recurrent hemorrhage.[8] The changes in CSF following hemorrhage are summarized in Table 1–8.

Table 1–8.   Changes in Cerebrospinal Fluid Following Hemorrhage*

Gross Examination

2–12 hours:	pink to orange xanthochromia
12–24 hours:	yellow xanthochromia (disappears in 2–4 weeks)

Microscopic Examination

2–24 hours:	erythrocytes, neutrophilic granulocytes (30%–60%), mononuclear phagocytes, lymphocytes
12–48 hours:	mononuclear phagocytes, erythrophagocytosis, lymphocytes
48 hours:	mononuclear phagocytes, erythrophagocytosis, siderophages (may persist for 2–8 weeks)

*Data adapted from Oehmichen.[8] Used by permission.

Lipophages or macrophages containing fat may be seen in traumatic or liquefaction necrosis associated with cerebral infarcts, and following myelography (Fig 17). Macrophages may also be observed in the CSF following pneumoencephalography, intrathecal therapy, and irradiation of the brain.[8]

Neutrophils may be seen in increased numbers in a variety of infectious and noninfectious disorders of the CNS (Table 1–9). The cytoplasmic granules of the PMNs are often less prominent than in the blood and show rapid disintegration upon standing (Figs 18 and 19).[7, 8] The latter may result in an inaccurate differential cell count.

Eosinophils are rarely seen in normal CSF. Increased numbers of eosinophils have been described in a variety of infectious and noninfectious disorders (Table 1–10) (Fig 20).[12] So-called idiopathic eosinophilic meningitis without evidence of a pathogen has also been described.[13]

Table 1–9. Causes of Cerebrospinal Fluid Neutrophilic Pleocytosis*

Bacterial meningitis
Early viral meningoencephalitis
Early tuberculous and mycotic meningitis
Amebic encephalomyelitis
Aseptic meningitis
Cerebral abscess, subdural empyema
CNS hemorrhage
Cerebral infarct
Malignancies
Previous lumbar puncture
Myelography, pneumoencephalography
Intrathecal injection of drugs
*Data adapted from Krieg.[2] Used by permission.

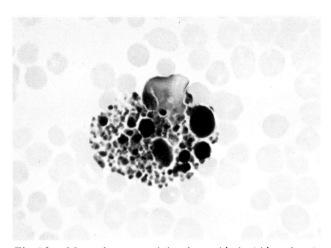

Fig 16. Macrophage containing hemosiderin (siderophage), demonstrated with an iron stain, from a patient with subarachnoid hemorrhage.

Table 1–10. Causes of Cerebrospinal Fluid Eosinophilic Pleocytosis*

Common
Parasitic infections
Fungal infections
Idiopathic eosinophilic meningitis
Reaction to foreign material in CNS (drugs, shunts)
Acute polyneuritis

Rare
Bacterial meningitis
Tuberculous meningoencephalitis
Viral meningitis
Leukemia, lymphoma
*Data adapted from Krieg.[2] Used by permission.

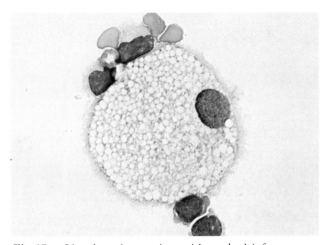

Fig 17. Lipophage in a patient with cerebral infarct.

Basophils are not seen in normal CSF but may be found in small numbers in a variety of abnormal conditions. Such conditions include inflammatory diseases, foreign body reactions, parasitic infections, convulsive disorders, and chronic granulocytic leukemia. Cases of basophilic meningitis associated with malignant lymphoma have been reported.[14]

Lupus erythematosus (LE) cells may rarely be seen in the CSF.[15]

Malignant cells from a variety of neoplasms may be encountered in the CSF.[16, 17] A CSF examination is particularly valuable in the diagnosis of metastatic carcinoma, leukemic and lymphomatous involvement of the meninges, and certain primary CNS tumors. Of the primary CNS tumors, medulloblastoma is more likely

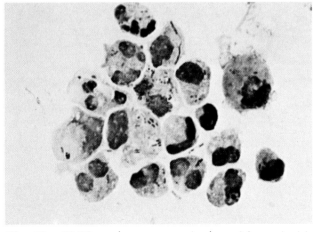

Fig 18. PMNs and monocytes in bacterial meningitis showing degenerative changes and poor staining characteristics.

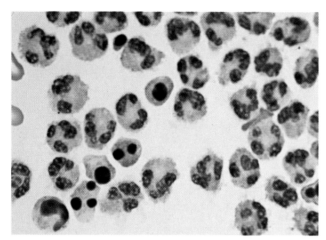

Fig 19. Neutrophilic pleocytosis with several degenerated and pyknotic neutrophils as seen in bacterial meningitis. The cells with pyknotic nuclei may be mistaken for nucleated RBCs.

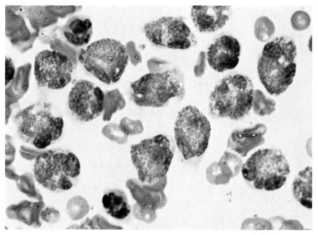

Fig 20. Eosinophilic pleocytosis in a patient with intracranial shunt.

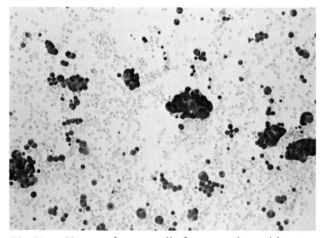

Fig 21. Clumps of tumor cells from a patient with metastatic oat cell carcinoma of the lung.

to be associated with malignant cells in the CSF than gliomas and meningiomas.[7, 8] When cells from metastatic tumors are detected in the CNS, melanoma and carcinoma of the lung (Figs 21 and 22), breast (Fig 23), and gastrointestinal tract are the most common.[7, 8] Malignant cells in the CSF may occur singly or more frequently in clumps. Clumps of ependymal cells or choroid plexus cells (see Figs 4 and 5), atypical lymphoid cells, and macrophages may be mistaken occasionally for tumor cells.

Clinical Correlations

In *bacterial meningitis,* the leukocyte count may be higher than 50,000/µl; more than 90% of these leukocytes are neutrophils in the early stages of the disease (Fig 24). In the very early stages of meningococcal meningitis, however, as few as 10% PMNs may be present. In addition to neutrophils, lymphocytes, monocytes, and macrophages are seen in moderate numbers. Successful treatment with antibiotics is usually associated with the rapid disappearance of neutrophils, while monocytes and macrophages become more prominent. Pathogenic organisms are often identified using a Gram's stain (Figs 25 and 26). Occasionally, leukocytosis of the CSF may persist despite successful antibiotic therapy. Such persistent pleocytosis is particularly associated with *Hemophilus influenzae* meningitis.[18]

Viral meningitis may be associated with mild or severe leukocytosis, predominantly composed of lymphocytes. It is important to note, however, that neutrophils may predominate initially (Fig 27). This granulocytic phase may last from a few hours to several days. Many different types of medium-sized and large, reactive lymphocytes are encountered (Fig 28). The large, reactive lymphocytes must be differentiated from lymphoblasts seen in *acute lymphoblastic leukemia (ALL).* In ALL, the lymphoblasts are generally uniform in size, shape, and appearance; while many different types of lymphocytes are present in reactive lymphocytosis. In the later stages of viral meningitis, lymphocytes decrease in number, while monocytes and macrophages become more evident.

Approximately 80% of the patients with untreated ALL and approximately 60% of the patients with *acute myelogenous leukemia (AML)* have leukemic cells in the CSF at some stage of the disease (Figs 29 and 30).

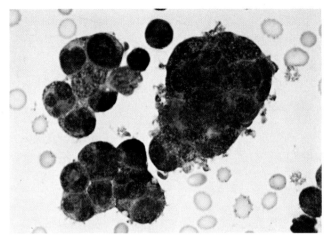

Fig 22. Metastatic oat cell carcinoma showing characteristic molding of nuclei.

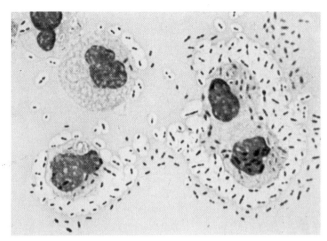

Fig 25. Bacterial meningitis with multiple organisms.

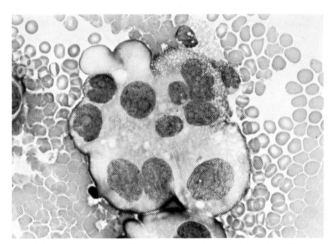

Fig 23. Malignant cells with indistinct cell borders from a patient with metastatic breast carcinoma.

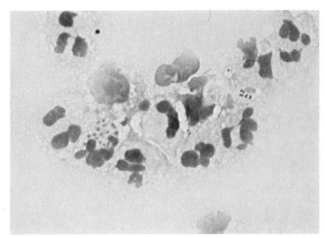

Fig 26. The presence of pathogenic organisms in the CSF *(Neisseria meningitidis)*, a characteristic finding in bacterial meningitis (Gram's stain).

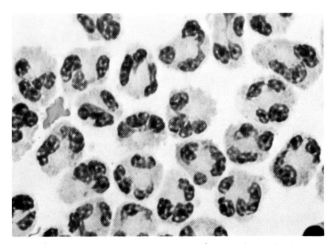

Fig 24. Neutrophilic pleocytosis in bacterial meningitis.

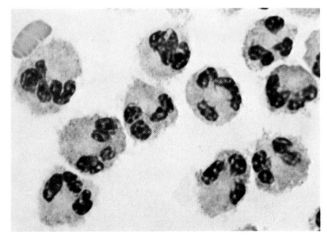

Fig 27. Neutrophilic pleocytosis in the early stage of viral meningitis.

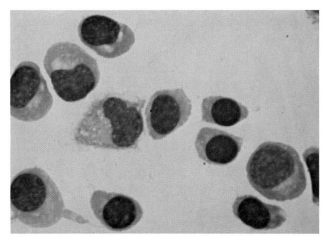

Fig 28. Different types of lymphocytes seen in a patient with viral meningitis.

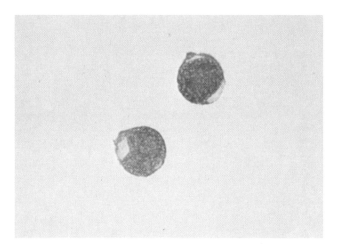

Fig 29. Lymphoblasts in a patient with acute lymphoblastic leukemia.

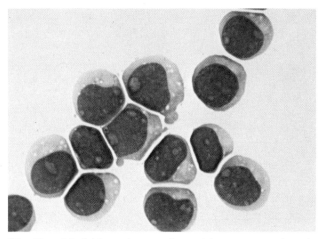

Fig 30. Myeloblasts in a patient with acute granulocytic leukemia.

Therefore, the CSF should be examined in all patients with acute leukemia.[19-21] The treatment of ALL now includes skull irradiation combined with intrathecal chemotherapy or intrathecal drugs alone.

When many lymphoblasts are present in the smear, there is usually no difficulty in making a correct diagnosis. The uniformity of the leukemic cells is the characteristic feature (Fig 31). However, when only a few cells are present, it may be extremely difficult to distinguish leukemic cells from atypical or transformed lymphocytes, or sometimes from atypical monocytes. It should be emphasized that an elevated CSF leukocyte count does not necessarily mean that leukemia is present, nor does a normal cell count exclude leukemic infiltration.[19, 20] The presence of an occasional lymphoblast is not limited to leukemia; as aforementioned, viral, bacterial, and fungal meningitis may be associated with lymphoblast-like cells in the CSF. Irradiation of the brain and intrathecal chemotherapy may also be associated with atypical mononuclear cells. The CSF may be contaminated with peripheral blood during the puncture and, occasionally, bone marrow may be aspirated from puncture of a vertebral body. A false-positive diagnosis of leukemia may be avoided if the diagnosis of leukemia is made in the presence of an increased total cell count, and when immature or abnormal cells constitute at least 40%–60% of the total cell population.[19] To make a correct diagnosis of leukemia, it is essential for the specimen to be adequate (> 2 ml), and the cells must be well preserved.[22] Finally, cytochemical studies using peroxidase and esterase stains may be helpful in the diagnosis. A careful correlation of clinical and cytologic findings is essential.

Small cell carcinoma of the lung (oat cell carcinoma) may be differentiated from acute leukemia by the former's tendency to form cell clusters and by the presence of more cytoplasm (see Fig 21). Medulloblastoma and metastatic neuroblastoma cells resemble lymphoblasts, but clustering of cells with nuclear molding by adjacent cells and rosette formation are typical of these tumors.[19]

Leptomeningeal involvement has been reported in 5%–27% of the patients with diffuse *non-Hodgkin's lymphoma* (Fig 32).[23, 24] The most common types are lymphoblastic lymphoma, diffuse histiocytic lymphoma (Fig 33), and undifferentiated lymphoma. Involvement of the CNS in nodular lymphomas is uncommon. It has been suggested that lymphoma cells spread directly from the medullary cavity along tissue planes through the dura and subarachnoid space.[23] A cytologic determination of the CSF is the most useful test for diagnosis and for monitoring response to therapy.

Iatrogenic conditions should also be considered when making diagnoses based on laboratory examination of the CSF. When a lumbar puncture has been repeated 8–12 hours after the initial puncture, the CSF may contain increased numbers of neutrophils, monocytes, macrophages, and occasional macrophages showing erythrophagocytosis.[8]

Pneumonencephalography and myelography may lead to pleocytosis consisting of lymphocytes, neutrophils, monocytes, macrophages, and eosinophils in varying numbers. An increased number of monocytes and macrophages may be present for 2–3 weeks following the procedure.[8]

Intracranial shunts for hydrocephalus may be associated with monocytosis and increased numbers of macrophages and eosinophils (see Fig 20).[8] The eosinophilic pleocytosis, particularly, may be quite striking and may represent an allergic reaction to the shunt.

Chemical Analysis

Protein

The CSF contains less than 1% of the amount of protein found in plasma. The normal concentration of lumbar CSF total protein is most often quoted as 15–45 mg/dl. However, these figures are not rigid, and reliable reference intervals vary considerably, depending on the method of analysis. As a result, an upper range of 40–60 mg/dl has been reported. In addition, age is an important variable. Newborns have relatively high values and compare with adult levels only after about 3–6 months. A recent study, involving high-risk neonates without meningitis, showed mean levels of 90 mg/dl for term infants and 115 mg/dl for preterm infants, with an upper range of 170 mg/dl.[3] Although the reasons for these high levels are not fully known, altered permeability of the blood-CSF barrier is the favored explanation. The total protein slowly increases after the age of 40 to a normal range of 30–60 mg/dl for 60 years and over.[2, 25] These figures refer only to spinal fluid removed through a lumbar puncture. Cisternal and ventricular fluids have lower levels of total protein.[2]

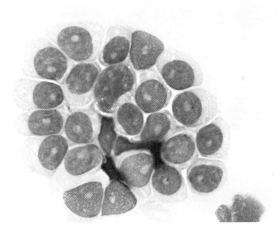

Fig 31. Prolymphocytes with characteristically prominent nucleoli in a patient with prolymphocytic leukemia. Note the uniformity of the cells.

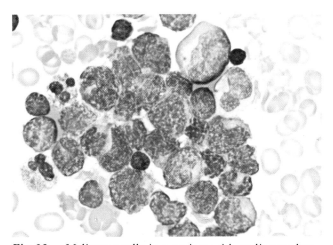

Fig 32. Malignant cells in a patient with malignant lymphoma, poorly differentiated lymphocytic type.

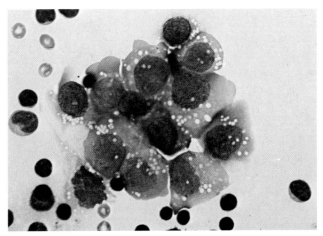

Fig 33. Malignant lymphoma, diffuse histiocytic type.

Elevation of the total protein is the most frequent pathologic finding in spinal fluid examination. Its elevation is nonspecific, but indicative of meningeal or CNS disease. Hence, elevations are seen in inflammatory processes, tumors, degenerative disorders, subarachnoid hemorrhage, and traumatic taps.[2] Mild elevations have also been reported with long-term administration of certain drugs, particularly the phenothiazines.

Levels of CSF protein below 15 mg/dl have been reported in some normal children older than 6 months of age, cases of water intoxication associated with increased intracranial pressure, and some leukemic patients. Low CSF protein levels have also been associated with CSF leakage from a dural tear, CSF rhinorrhea or otorrhea, hyperthyroidism, and some instances in which large amounts of fluid have been removed for pneumoencephalography and the CSF is diluted from the cisterna magna.[2]

Accurate determination of spinal fluid protein is hampered by several factors including its low concentration, the presence of different types of protein (mainly albumin and globulin), and the small amount of fluid usually available for analysis. Many different methods have been used for its quantitative estimation. The most common methods in use are turbidimetric procedures involving agents such as sulfosalicylic acid. These procedures are popular since they are rapid, easily performed, and use instruments that are readily available. They are reasonably accurate but are deficient in that albumin gives about four times more turbidity than a comparable amount of globulin.[26] Another problem with these methods is that there is a linear relationship between temperature and turbidity; hence, reasonably constant temperature control is essential. Methods that combine sulfosalicylic acid and sodium sulfate, or use trichloroacetic acid (TCA), react with albumin and globulin more equally. Albumin should not be used as a standard when using turbidometric methods.[26]

Some of the same difficulties are encountered in most of the colorimetric techniques. In addition, there is another problem—the reagent used often reacts with nonprotein nitrogenous substances. Although the Lowry method[27] is least affected by varying albumin-globulin ratios, a serious drawback is the interference from nonprotein compounds.

Theoretically, spectrophotometry at 210–220 nm has several desirable attributes including high sensitivity; similar absorption for albumin and globulin, since it is the peptide bond that absorbs at this wavelength; and small sample requirement. The major problem with the direct measurement is the interference of other substances such as nucleosides, nucleotides, ascorbic acid, various carboxylic acids, and drugs that also absorb light in this range. The use of prior gel filtration of the CSF eliminates these interferences to provide a highly reliable and valuable technique.[28, 29] Normal values are a little higher than with other methods (upper limits of the reference interval = 60 mg/dl), but the precision is better. The only real drawback appears to be the need for high quality instrumentation that is reliable at 210–220 nm.

Other less commonly used methods include the modified biuret, dye binding, and immunologic procedures. A relatively recent and unique colorimetric micromethod has been published.[30] This method is based on the coprecipitation of protein and ponceau S dye by TCA, dissolution of the precipitate in weak alkali, and readings made at 560 nm. The method is independent of temperature, relatively unaffected by the albumin-globulin ratio, and appears not to react with nonprotein substances. Although it gives lower values than either the Lowry or TCA methods, it correlates well with the reference Kjeldahl technique.

Protein Fractionation

The fractionation of spinal fluid protein may be of considerable value in certain disorders. Most of the proteins present in normal serum have also been demonstrated in CSF. These include prealbumin, albumin, transferrin, fibrinogen, ceruloplasmin, haptoglobulins, α_2-macroglobulin, IgG, IgA, and others. Most of these substances are derived from plasma. Their relative concentrations correlate well with the hydrodynamic radii and less with the molecular weights of the protein components. Some proteins, mainly the γ-globulins, can be produced within the CNS.

Spinal fluid proteins can be separated by electrophoresis using paper, cellulose acetate, agarose, and polyacrylamide gel.[2] The major defined fractions include prealbumin, albumin, α_1-globulin, α_2-globulin, β-globulin including the τ-fraction, and γ-globulin. The τ-fraction, which represents a carbohydrate-deficient form of transferrin, is less conspicuous when the protein has not been denatured. Although fractionation studies have been conducted on unconcentrated fluid, it is recommended that the CSF be concentrated prior to electrophoresis. Many types of concentration techniques have been used[31-33] and have yielded reasonably similar reference values (Table 1-11).

Using paper electrophoresis, Ivers et al[34] found that the CSF of 72% of 144 patients with multiple sclerosis (MS) had increased γ-globulin levels. Many of these patients had a normal total protein. This study has been repeatedly verified. However, the finding of an elevated γ-globulin is not specific for this disease. Similar increases may be found in a variety of acute infections, neurosyphilis, subacute panencephalitis, Guillain-Barré syndrome, meningeal carcinomatosis, and other neurologic conditions. It should also be noted that patients with cirrhosis, sarcoidosis, myxedema, collagen vascular disorders, multiple myeloma, and other conditions that are associated with increased levels of serum γ-globulin may also have increased levels of CSF γ-globulin. Hence, a serum electrophoretic pattern may be imperative to interpret the CSF study properly. Furthermore, it should be emphasized that it is the percentage of γ-globulin that is of major diagnostic significance, and not its absolute value.

When agarose or agar gel is used, in contrast to paper or cellulose acetate, the γ-globulins in spinal fluid from patients with MS migrate as discrete populations forming so-called *oligoclonal bands*.[35, 36] These abnormal patterns have been noted in 90% or more of the patients with clinically active MS, making agar gel electrophoresis the single most sensitive and reliable method currently available for the diagnosis of this disorder.[36] However, this finding is not specific for MS, since disorders that show increased CSF γ-globulins may also have oligoclonal bands. Oligoclonal bands in the CSF may not indicate MS if similar bands are present in the serum. It is advised that serum electrophoresis also be done in agar in these instances.[2]

Immunoglobulins

As indicated previously, the CSF proteins are derived either by diffusion across the blood-CSF barrier or by synthesis within the CNS. The normal plasma to CSF ratio for albumin is about 230.[2] The plasma to CSF IgG ratio is less well established with values reported to be 370-800.[25, 37] The plasma to CSF albumin ratio is decreased with a traumatic tap, increased blood-CSF permeability, or impaired resorption. The plasma to CSF IgG ratio reflects both synthesis of IgG in the CNS and the blood-CNS barrier, and blood-CSF permeability.

Kabat et al,[38] using the classic Tiselius technique for electrophoresis, were the first to note that the CSF γ-globulin was increased in patients with neurosyphilis and MS. Approximately 75% of the patients with MS have increased CSF γ-globulins when expressed as a percentage of CSF total protein or CSF albumin.[2] Kabat and others[39] later developed an immunochemical method for CSF immunoglobulin quantitation that still serves as the reference technique. However, this method is too tedious for routine clinical work; and it was not until 1966 that the process of electroimmunodiffusion (EID), suitable for use with small quantities of unconcentrated CSF, was described by Hartley et al.[40] This technique made it possible to study CSF immunoglobulins routinely and to establish reliable refer-

Table 1-11.   Reference Values for Electrophoresis of Cerebrospinal Fluid Proteins*

Protein	Source		
	Kaplan ($\bar{x} \pm SD$, %)	Windisch and Bracken ($\bar{x} \pm SD$, %)	Breebaart et al† (mg/dl $\pm$ 2SD)
Prealbumin	4.9 ± 1.2	3.8 ± 1.18	0.4-2.5
Albumin	61.5 ± 5.3	65.5 ± 5.34	7.0-34.0
α_1-globulin	4.5 ± 1.4	3.6 ± 1.32	0.7-3.6
α_2-globulin	6.7 ± 1.8	6.8 ± 2.15	0.9-4.0
β-globulin	13.7 ± 3.6	12.4 ± 2.62	1.9-7.5
γ-globulin	8.8 ± 2.6	7.6 ± 2.36	0.7-4.3

*Data adapted from Kaplan,[31] Windisch and Bracken,[32] and Breebaart et al.[33]
†Study focused on subjects 20-40 years of age. The γ-globulin was slightly higher after age 40.

ence values for IgG and possibly IgA in unconcentrated CSF; nonetheless, IgM could not be detected in unconcentrated fluid. They also noted that the concentration of spinal fluid resulted in considerable destruction of the immunoglobulins, particularly IgG. A comparison of normal protein fractions in serum and CSF is illustrated in Table 1–12.

Table 1–12.   Comparison of Approximate Normal Protein Fractions in Cerebrospinal Fluid and Serum

Protein	CSF (mg/dl)	Serum (mg/dl)
Total protein	15–45	6,000–8,000
Albumin	10–30	3,500–5,000
IgG	0.7–4.0	800–1,500
IgA	0–0.4	90–450
IgM	0	6–250

In recent years two additional techniques, radial immunodiffusion (RID) and nephelometry, have been introduced to measure IgG and albumin in the CSF. In RID, the antigen being assayed diffuses radially through agar gel containing monospecific antiserum to that protein. A precipitin ring forms when the antigen-antibody complex approaches equivalence. The concentration of the antigen is proportional to the square of the diameter of the precipitin ring.

Nephelometry is a quantitative determination of turbidity by measuring light scattering. Immunoglobulins are quantitated by measuring either the rate of formation of the antigen-antibody complex or the total amount of complex. A recent report comparing RID with nephelometry showed that RID had greater precision in measuring both IgG and albumin.[41] The nephelometric techniques, however, are much more rapid and convenient. Results are available within 1–60 minutes, depending on the system used.

Although the measurement of IgA and IgM is possible, at present it has no clinical usefulness. Total IgG is also of little help. However, when IgG is expressed as a percentage of the CSF total protein, or more accurately as a percentage of albumin, since albumin is more precisely measured, valuable information can be obtained. Approximately 75% of the patients with MS will have an elevated ratio using CSF total protein or CSF albumin. Unfortunately, reported normal ratios

vary considerably, probably due to the use of different standards and antisera.

Reliable interpretation of these ratios is possible if one considers the upper limits to be 10.5% for IgG/total protein and 25%–28% for IgG/albumin in normal CSF.[37] The importance of these ratios over absolute IgG measurements is that they "correct" for increased IgG in the CSF due to increased permeability of the blood-CSF barrier and provide evidence that the increased IgG is from local production within the CNS.

A more sophisticated, recommended method of correction to allow for changes in the plasma proteins as well as for increased CSF-blood barrier permeability is the *IgG/albumin index.*[25]

$$\text{IgG/albumin index} = \frac{\text{CSF IgG/plasma IgG}}{\text{CSF albumin/plasma albumin}}$$

The normal range for this index is 0.34–0.58 (mean ± 2SD). About 85% of patients with MS have an increased IgG/albumin index.[25]

Link and Zetterwall quantitated the CSF immunoglobulin κ and λ light chains.[42] They pointed out that patients with MS may have IgG with an abnormal light chain distribution, most commonly an increase in the κ to λ ratio. Similar studies have been reported by Palmer et al.[43] These findings need further clinical evaluation, however, before their full significance is known.

In MS, leukodystrophies, and other demyelinating syndromes, the myelin sheaths are selectively degraded. Demyelination can also occur as a secondary disorder in various intoxications, infections, vascular lesions, and other conditions. In these secondary disorders, not only myelin but other CNS components (eg, nerve cells and axons) are also degraded. In all these conditions, myelin basic protein is released and appears in the CSF where it can be accurately detected using radioimmunoassay.[44] The antiserum is produced by inoculating rabbits with guinea pig spinal cord that has been homogenized in complete Freund adjuvant. Assays are done on duplicate 0.5 ml samples of the CSF, and results are reported as negative (< 4 ng/ml), weakly positive (4–8 ng/ml), or positive (> 8 ng/ml). Elevated levels have been found in patients with MS during exacerbations of the disease, while no myelin basic protein has been found during remission. It should be emphasized, however, that the assay for myelin basic protein is not specific for MS and should not be used as a definitive test for MS. Nonetheless, the test may be a useful indicator of active demyelination.

Glucose

Specimens submitted for glucose analysis should be run without delay. Normal levels of glucose in the CSF are approximately 60%–70% of plasma values, the generally accepted range being 50–80 mg/dl in the fasting state.[2] Glucose levels in the 40–45 mg/dl range are considered equivocal. This range assumes a normal fasting serum of 65–100 mg/dl and is based on the use of highly specific methods for glucose analysis. A "bloody tap" will, of course, cause a false elevation.

Glucose enters the CSF from plasma by two major mechanisms—diffusion and active transport. The former is influenced by the concentration and duration of the plasma glucose level. Hence, changes in plasma glucose levels are not seen in the CSF until 30–90 minutes later. For this reason, it is preferable to analyze the plasma level at least 30 minutes before determining the CSF value. Otherwise, an inaccurate interpretation may result.

An elevated CSF glucose, either absolute or relative to the plasma glucose, is evidence of hyperglycemia 0.5–2.0 hours prior to obtaining the specimen. It has no specific significance unless the patient is diabetic, and the CSF glucose is less than about 40%–50% of the plasma value.

Decreased glucose values, classically seen in bacterial and tuberculous (or fungal) meningitis, may also be present in a variety of other conditions such as hypoglycemia, primary or metastatic tumor involving the meninges, and subarachnoid hemorrhage due to the release of glycolytic enzymes from RBCs. Occasionally decreased levels are found in viral meningitis, but they are more frequently normal. Other conditions such as a brain abscess and neurosyphilis are usually associated with normal glucose levels.

There are several mechanisms to explain low spinal fluid glucose in bacterial meningitis. The initial mechanism proposed was glucose utilization by bacteria, a theory now known to be untenable in terms of the amount of glucose that can be metabolized by bacteria. A second proposal, the utilization of glucose by phagocytizing neutrophils, while true to some extent, has two major objections. In the first place, it fails to explain the low CSF glucose levels seen in tuberculous meningitis where mononuclear cells predominate and few organisms are present. Secondly, maximal glucose utilization by leukocytes is small in comparison to the amount used by the brain. It is argued that the major

explanation for increased glucose utilization in bacterial meningitis is defective glucose transport and increased glycolytic activity in the brain.[45]

Although decreased CSF glucose levels in bacterial meningitis are commonly seen, it is not unusual to find normal values when cultures are positive. In their classic series of articles on bacterial meningitis involving 207 patients, Swartz and Dodge[46] reported low levels in only 55% of the cases of pneumococcal meningitis, 53% of the meningitis cases caused by *Hemophilus influenzae,* and 45% of the meningococcal meningitis cases. Other studies suggest that CSF glucose is decreased in a higher percentage of cases, especially in children, where low levels are seen in 60%–80% of the cases.[47]

Direct comparisons between glucose and lactate in the CSF have not been specifically reported, but published data suggest that elevated lactate levels are more frequently seen than decreased glucose levels in bacterial meningitis.[48] Our own initial data involving 47 consecutive cases of bacterial meningitis in children, 40 of which were caused by *H influenzae,* showed levels of lactate greater than 30 mg/dl in 100% of the cases. Glucose levels less than 40 mg/dl were seen in 83% (39 of the 47 cases studied).

The glucose oxidase test strips have for a long time been considered useful in distinguishing CSF from nasal secretions. Several studies have, however, shown that this test is of no clinical value.[49] Glucose can be demonstrated in most samples of nasal discharge, and the diagnosis of CSF rhinorrhea or otorrhea must be made by other methods such as intrathecal ^{131}I serum albumin.[2]

Enzymes

Many studies have been conducted in an attempt to relate evaluations of various enzymes with diseases involving the CNS. Yet, despite frequent abnormalities, this field of study remains somewhat clouded as to the value of these assays and how well they correlate with the diagnosis of various neurologic disorders. The topic has been recently reviewed.[50]

The clinical implications of *lactate dehydrogenase (LD)* assays of the CSF were first reported in 1958.[51] It was demonstrated that the CSF levels of LD varied independently of plasma activity; and that patients with CNS leukemia, lymphoma, metastatic carcinoma, and subarachnoid hemorrhage had consistently elevated values when compared with controls. In addition, marked increases occurred in acute meningitis and returned to normal after successful treatment. Subsequent studies not only confirmed these findings but showed that the LD assays were helpful in differentiating acute bacterial from viral meningitis. While the latter condition is usually associated with normal to mildly elevated LD activity,[52] partially treated cases of bacterial meningitis usually show increased levels.

One of the primary problems in evaluating CSF specimens has been the lack of reliable reference values for many analytes, since large volumes of normal fluid are difficult to obtain. This problem is further complicated by enzyme analysis, since methodologies vary greatly and values change with substrate, buffer, and reaction conditions. As a result, reliable normal values on an adequate control population, using quality kinetic spectrophotometric assays, are not available. The data of Wroblewski and associates suggest that normal plasma LD levels are 15 to 20 times higher than those seen in the CSF.[51] A relatively recent study, using reliable methodology but with a modest number of controls, reported a "normal range" of 3–17 units/liter at 30 C.[53] The corresponding normal plasma levels were not given. In the same study, cases of bacterial meningitis and CNS leukemia almost invariably had enzyme activities greater than 3.0 times the upper limit of the normal range, while those cases with other tumors and viral infections had levels less than 2.5 times this upper limit.

It is important to remember that a "bloody tap" or fluid showing a recent or old hemorrhage will have markedly abnormal LD levels. The RBCs contain 100 to 150 times the LD concentration of plasma, and plasma contains 15 to 20 times the LD activity of the CSF.

By appropriate CSF concentration, *LD isoenzymes* can be readily studied. This technique has increased the specificity of enzyme analysis.[53, 54] These reports have shown that the normal CSF isoenzyme distribution is $LD_1 > LD_2 > LD_3 > LD_4 > LD_5$, with the latter two isoenzymes being no more than a small percentage of the total. Brain tissue, which is rich in LD, has a similar isoenzyme distribution but is more closely related to normal plasma with a reversal of isoenzymes LD_1 and LD_2, ie, $LD_2 > LD_1$. Consequently, various neurologic disorders (hydrocephalus, increased intracranial pressure, and chronic epilepsy) that have mild elevations of total LD show a "normal" distribution.

In bacterial meningitis, the isoenzyme pattern is usually the exact opposite of normal CSF with $LD_5 > LD_4 > LD_3 > LD_2 > LD_1$. Although some cases vary slightly, LD_5 is invariably the dominant isoenzyme. Isoenzymes LD_4 and LD_5 predominate in granulocytes and are presumed to be the major enzyme source. In viral meningitis, the isoenzyme pattern is usually a combination of that seen in the brain and lymphocytes, ie, $LD_2 > LD_1 > LD_3$ or $LD_2 > LD_3 > LD_1$; lymphocytes contain predominately LD_2 and LD_3. High levels of LD_1 and LD_2 in viral and bacterial meningitis are thought to be associated with severe CNS damage and a poor prognosis.[2] In CNS childhood leukemia (acute lymphoblastic), the distribution of isoenzymes is essentially that of purified lymphoblasts, the major components being $LD_4 > LD_3 > LD_5$.

These studies of the clinical implications of isoenzyme distribution look promising, but to fully evaluate the usefulness of total LD and its isoenzymes in disorders of the CNS, reliable reference intervals need to be established and compared to other variables.

Like LD, *aspartate aminotransferase (AST or GOT)* is normally present in the CSF but in smaller quantities than its serum counterpart. Again, reliable reference intervals are not available for the same reasons expressed for LD. The AST levels increase with age. As with LD, one must be careful in evaluating enzyme activities performed on "bloody taps" or xanthochromic fluid, since AST is about ten times more concentrated in RBCs than in plasma, and plasma has more activity than spinal fluid.

The CSF and serum AST levels vary independently of each other. Increased AST levels in the CSF have been noted in some brain tumors, cerebral infarction, and contusion (but not concussion); elevated values have also occurred within 48 hours of seizure activity in adults and after CNS radiation and/or chemotherapy. They have not been found to be consistently elevated in inflammatory processes.

Overall, the AST measurement has not been very helpful as an aid in the evaluation of CNS disorders. As a result, its clinical usefulness, if any, must await further studies.

Creatine kinase (CK or CPK) is normally present in brain tissue, along with skeletal muscle and myocardium, where it is thought to participate in maintaining adequate supplies of ATP. It is not present in RBCs.

Elevated CK levels have been reported with some

discrepancies in acute subarachnoid hemorrhage, hydrocephalus, cerebral infarction, muscular dystrophy, brain tumors, and conditions associated with increased intracranial pressure. In addition, its degree of elevation may have some value in facilitating the prognosis in cases of head trauma.[55] Data indicating its elevation in acute psychosis appear contradictory.

The measurement of CK isoenzymes would appear to be more useful, since the brain contains almost 100% of the isoenzyme, CK_1 (BB). Nevertheless, neither an elevated total CK nor an isoenzyme profile has been shown to be particularly useful in clinical conditions except possibly as an early aid in differentiating mild from moderate brain trauma.

Lysozyme (muramidase) is a low molecular weight protein (mol wt about 15,000) that actively catalyzes the breakdown of mucopolysaccharides in bacterial cell walls. The lysozyme concentration is very high in neutrophils and monocytes. It is also present in considerable quantities in the gastrointestinal tract and kidneys.

In normal persons, the lysozyme concentration in the CSF is either absent or barely detectable. The highest values are seen in acute bacterial meningitis. The levels appear to correlate both with the CSF protein concentration and the number of neutrophilic leukocytes.[56] As a result, the CSF lysozyme is usually normal in viral meningitis. Elevated levels have also been reported in cerebrovascular disease, MS, intracranial hemorrhage, and epilepsy. High concentrations would be expected in cases of acute myelomonoblastic and acute monocytic leukemia or histiocytic lymphoma when these disorders affect the CNS. In most tumors of the CNS, the enzyme is apparently directly related to protein concentration. When a CSF cytologic study shows no abnormalities and protein levels are normal, the lysozyme concentration is also normal.[57] It appears that lysozyme has negligible value as a specific aid in the diagnosis of CNS tumors.

Several other enzymes have been measured in the CSF in an attempt to correlate their activities with various disease processes. These include ribonuclease, cholinesterase, arginine esterase, adenylate kinase, and dopamine-β-hydroxylase, among others. At this time, more research is needed to fully evaluate the potential usefulness of these enzymes in CNS disorders.

Amino Compounds

Increased levels of *ammonia* in the CSF are seen in a variety of liver diseases that lead to hepatic encephalopathy, including Reye's syndrome in children. In addition, elevated values occur in hypercapnea.[58] In all these conditions, elevated CSF levels appear to correlate with the degree of encephalopathy. Normal CSF values of ammonia are about one half that of blood levels.

Several investigators have also shown that *glutamine* correlates well with the severity of hepatic encephalopathy. This compound is synthesized by the brain from ammonia and glutamic acid and provides the means whereby ammonia is removed from the CNS. However, as more ammonia and glutamic acid react, other intermediates of cerebral metabolism, such as α-ketoglutarate, become depleted. This loss of critical metabolic intermediates may be one of the contributing factors in the development of hepatic encephalopathy.

The CSF concentration of glutamine is increased in about 75% of the patients with Reye's syndrome.[59] Normal values of CSF constituents, eg, ammonia, depend on the methodology used. When glutamine is deaminated with sulfuric acid, and the liberated ammonia is measured by either Nessler's reagent or phenolhypochlorite,[60, 61] the upper limit of the normal range is approximately 20 mg/dl. When ammonia is measured enzymatically, the upper boundary of the normal scope is 15 mg/dl.[2]

The *biogenic amines* (5-hydroxytryptamine, norepinephrine, and dopamine) have been suggested as synaptic transmitters in the CNS.[62] Each amine is thought to function in a distinct system of the brain: 5-hydroxytryptamine (serotonin, 5-HT) in the limbic structures, norepinephrine in the central autonomic system, and dopamine in the extra pyramidal system. These compounds are formed from precursor aromatic amino acids that enter the brain from the blood, become ring-hydroxylated, and then are decarboxylated to form the specific aromatic amine.

Although these substances cannot be directly measured in the CSF, some of their metabolites can, such as 5-hydroxyindoleacetic acid (5-HIAA) from 5-HT and homovanillic acid (HVA) from dopamine. On the other hand, in contrast to that seen in the peripheral nervous system, vanillylmandelic acid is apparently not the end product of norepinephrine metabolism. The major product here is unknown, although 3-methoxy-4-hydroxy phenylethylene glycol and vanillic acid are both found in the CSF and are presumably derived through this pathway.

The measurement of these metabolites in CSF, especially HVA and 5-HIAA, has been thought to provide an index of disease. In part, this appears to be true, inasmuch as the concentrations of both 5-HIAA and HVA have been shown to be significantly decreased in both the caudate nucleus and lateral ventricular fluid from patients with Parkinson's disease. This finding may be more difficult to demonstrate in CSF taken from the lumbar sac, since the fluid here is not homogeneous. Certain rules must be followed in sampling from this site to obtain reproducible data.[63]

Various other metabolites in the CSF have been reported recently. It appears that palmitic acid is present in normal CSF in the greatest concentration of any organic acid.[64] Stearic acid is also prominently present. In one study, significant amounts of 3-methoxy-4-hydroxyphenyl ethanol were found in 28 of 37 samples of normal fluid.[64] The clinical significance, if any, of measuring these compounds will have to await further investigations.

Other amines and amino acids have been measured in the CSF. One compound of possible significance is the report of increased amounts of *ethanolamine* in the CSF of autistic children.[65] It appears possible that a subgroup of these children may have a brain disorder related to the abnormal metabolism of this compound.

Elevated concentrations of *glycine* in plasma are seen in a wide variety of metabolic disorders. Two of these disorders, albeit very rare, are most easily detected by appropriate analysis of the CSF. The first of these is nonketotic hyperglycinemia. In ketotic hyperglycinemia, plasma elevations of glycine appear to be secondary to the accumulation of one or more organic acids that are products of the branched-chain amino acids. Examples of these disorders include propionic acidemia, isovaleric acidemia, and methylmalonic acidemia.

Most children with nonketotic hyperglycinemia, however, have no apparent organic acid abnormality. This is a heterogeneous group of disorders, but in some cases, a severe illness develops early in childhood that usually leads to death. In these cases, but not in the ketotic ones, the CSF glycine levels are increased 15 to 30 times the normal level. The basic defect appears to be the absence of a glycine cleavage enzyme.[66]

Homocarnosinosis is a familial metabolic disorder, characterized by elevated *homocarnosine* (a dipeptide composed of γ-aminobutyric acid and histidine). In this disorder, the homocarnosine levels are 20 times that of normal controls.[67]

Although amines and amino acids are not measured routinely, and most of these measurements are currently of little practical value, they may prove to have considerable diagnostic value in the future.

Electrolytes

The measurement of CSF *sodium* is not considered to be clinically useful in the diagnosis of neurologic disorders. The levels of sodium found in the CSF parallel those found in serum but appear to fluctuate less in cases of hyponatremia and hypernatremia.

Reference intervals for CSF *potassium*, as determined by several groups of investigators, are consistently in the range of 2.6–3.1 mmole/liter,[68] a much lower and more narrow interval than for plasma (3.5–5.0 mmole/liter). There is essentially no fluctuation of CSF potassium with systemic acid-base abnormalities; hence, the routine measurement of CSF potassium has little clinical importance in these situations. On the other hand, significant changes in potassium have been reported in cisternal fluid following cardiac arrest and may give some indication of the degree of cerebral damage.[69] The potassium concentration increases in cisternal fluid following cardiac arrest. This increase is significantly greater in those patients who do not regain consciousness in comparison to those who do.

Unlike most other CSF constituents, CSF *chloride* is present in higher concentrations than in plasma, the normal range being approximately 115–130 mmole/liter. Plasma levels are quite labile, and changes are rapidly reflected in the CSF. As a result, any condition characterized by hypochloremia or hyperchloremia will show comparable changes in the CSF. In the past, determination of CSF chloride was thought to be helpful in the diagnosis of meningitis, particularly the tuberculous type in which decreased levels are consistently seen. This finding, however, merely reflects the hypochloremia usually seen in most patients with meningitis, regardless of the cause. Therefore, CSF chloride measurements are not considered to be of any current value in the diagnosis of meningitis or any other neurologic disorder.

Spinal fluid contains approximately one half the concentration of the total *calcium* in plasma and is essentially equal to the nonprotein-bound or diffusable calcium in plasma. Changes in ionized serum calcium are rapidly reflected in the CSF. Active transport is another operating mechanism.

In contrast to calcium, the CSF concentrations of *magnesium* are normally maintained at levels averaging

30% greater than those in serum. Patients with infectious diseases and apparently some with ischemic brain disease lose their ability to maintain this high concentration in the CSF.[70]

There appears to be no known clinical usefulness in the measurement of either calcium or magnesium in the CSF.

Acids and Bases

In 1917, Levinson first demonstrated that patients with acute bacterial meningitis have a decrease in the CSF pH.[71] More recently, this measurement, along with that of CSF lactate, has been shown to be helpful in the early diagnosis of bacterial meningitis,[72] although the laboratory value of CSF lactate is probably a more reliable indicator (see section entitled "Lactate").

In recent years, the measurements of pH, pCO_2, and bicarbonate in the CSF have received considerable attention.[73, 74] However, from a clinical standpoint, these CSF measurements are still in the experimental phase; yet, they may soon prove to be clinically useful. For example, the consistent finding that acute cerebral edema following head trauma is frequently preceded by a persistent reduction in CSF bicarbonate may provide helpful information in these cases.[75] Other conditions such as hypoxia and salicylate intoxication may prove to be more easily managed when these measurements are routinely available.

Lactate

The measurement of CSF lactate is now considered to be an important adjunct in the early differential diagnosis of viral vs bacterial meningitis.

Increased levels of CSF lactic acid in tuberculous and meningococcal meningitis were first noted by Nishimura in 1924. The general recognition of the clinical value of these findings, however, has only recently been realized.[76-79] These studies have uniformly supported Nishimura's observations. In addition, infections due to mycoplasma usually show increased levels of CSF lactate. Partially treated cases of bacterial meningitis generally have elevated levels as well. However, appropriate therapy leads to a rapid recovery. Patients with viral meningitis almost invariably have normal values, although occasional cases are associated with borderline or minimally elevated lactate levels.

The mechanism for elevated CSF lactate appears to be tissue hypoxia due to increased intracranial pressure with subsequent impairment of the central blood supply. Therefore, any condition associated with decreased blood flow or deficient oxygenation of the brain can cause increased lactate levels.[78] Such conditions include intracranial hemorrhage, brain abscess, cerebral arteriosclerosis, hypotension, low arterial CO_2, primary and metastatic malignancies, traumatic brain injuries, and idiopathic seizures.[2] Xanthochromic fluids invariably show high lactate levels originating from RBCs and should probably not be analyzed for lactate, since the results are usually misleading.

Lactate in the CSF is readily and accurately measured using either enzymatic or gas-liquid chromatographic techniques. They yield essentially identical results. Normal values are in the range of 10–25 mg/dl (1.11–2.81 mmole/liter).[80] Values in the 25–30 mg/dl range should be considered equivocal. Early diagnosed cases of bacterial meningitis may have values in the equivocal range, although the great majority exceed 30 mg/dl. On the other hand, lactate levels associated with cases of viral meningitis almost invariably fall below 25 mg/dl, although occasional cases have been reported with values in the equivocal range. Appropriate serologic tests must be carried out to identify infections due to mycoplasma. Cultures in these cases are negative, but lactate levels are usually elevated. If the serologic studies are deleted, one may mistake these for cases of viral meningitis with high values of lactate.

Other Biochemical Measurements

Urea, uric acid, zinc, phosphorus, ethanol, and various hormones, among other substances, have been measured in the spinal fluid; and reference values have been established. None of these measurements are considered to be of current clinical value except possibly for a few of the hormones.[2] In particular, the CSF measurement of adenohypophyseal hormones may be of value in diagnosing cases of extensions of pituitary tumors or in monitoring their therapeutic responses. In addition, human chorionic gonadotropin has been measured in the CSF for the detection of metastatic choriocarcinoma. These studies need further investigation.

Microbiologic Examination

Appropriate microbiologic examination is essential in every patient in whom the clinical findings suggest even the slightest possibility of meningitis. The major reasons for this are as follows: (1) Untreated bacterial meningitis is a lethal disease capable of rapid progression, (2) early treatment with appropriate antibiotic therapy is curative, and (3) the selection of adequate antimicrobics depends on the knowledge of a specific causative agent that often requires in vitro susceptibility testing.

The CSF should be cultured and a Gram's stain performed. In addition, blood cultures should be obtained since these will be positive in 40%–60% of the cases. Blood cultures may provide the only definitive clue as to the causative agent, inasmuch as CSF cultures will be positive in only 70%–90% of the cases. Routine cultures of the pharynx or external ear are not usually warranted and may be highly misleading, since the most common organisms causing meningitis are frequent inhabitants of these locations.

Fully 80%–90% of the cases of bacterial meningitis are caused by *H influenzae, Neisseria meningitidis,* and *Streptococcus pneumoniae.* The remaining 10%–20% of the cases are caused by *Staphylococcus aureus,* enteric organisms, and anaerobic and microaerophilic streptococci, which are often associated with epidural empyema, brain abscess, neurosurgical procedures, or head trauma. Rare cases of meningitis caused by *Listeria monocytogenes* (easily confused with diphtheroids) or *Mima-Herellea* (may resemble *H influenzae* or *N meningitidis*) may be seen.

H influenzae meningitis, encountered almost exclusively in children between 2 months and 6 years of age, comprises over 60% of the cases of postneonatal meningitis. In the neonatal period, the Enterobacteriaceae are the causative agents in 60%–70% of the cases. More specifically, *Escherichia coli* is isolated about 40% of the time.

A quality Gram's stain of the sedimented CSF, examined by an expert microbiologist, will yield an accurate, presumptive diagnosis in the majority of cases (perhaps up to 80%), although its reliability is probably considerably less than this in most institutions. The most common diagnostic errors are misinterpretating precipitated dye or stained debris for gram-positive organisms, stained nuclear fragments for gram-negative organisms, or dead bacteria in collection tubes. Compounding these problems with the Gram's stain have been the time delay for culture reports and the frequency of negative cultures. As a result, the measurement of CSF glucose and lactate has become more precise with the use of counterimmunoelectrophoresis (CIE) and the Limulus lysate test, thus accelerating the laboratory diagnosis of bacterial meningitis.

The hematogenous dissemination of tubercle bacilli to the brain and meninges may result in chronic meningitis or simulate an intracranial neoplasm. Children who have miliary tuberculosis at the time of primary infection are at greater risk of contracting CNS tuberculosis than adults who have the disease in a disseminated form. In suspected cases, an acid-fast stain of the sedimented CSF and appropriate cultures are needed. The number of organisms is usually small, and patience is needed in examination of the smears. The fluorescent rhodamine stain may be more sensitive than the Ziehl-Neelsen method.[2] Chemical determinations are frequently helpful as the CSF lactate will be elevated above 30 mg/dl, the glucose decreased below 35 mg/dl, and the protein increased in most cases. These findings, plus the presence of increased numbers of leukocytes, predominantly mononuclear, should certainly arouse suspicion that the case might be one of tuberculous meningitis.

Viral meningitis is caused by a variety of infectious agents. Those most commonly involved are the enteroviruses, mumps virus, and the arboviruses. Other occasional agents include herpes simplex virus and the lymphocytic choriomeningitis viruses. Adenoviruses and rhinoviruses are rarely implicated. An exact diagnosis requires special isolation techniques and serologic methods for a specific antibody. When these are used, a causative agent can be identified in approximately 70% of the cases. It is important to emphasize that the earlier in the clinical course that the specimen is collected, the more probable the virus will be identified. In these cases, viruses should also be sought in the feces (enteroviruses, herpes virus), urine (mumps), saliva (herpes virus and mumps), and throat washings (enteroviruses, lymphocytic choriomeningitis viruses, and herpes virus). Since viremia occurs prior to the onset of meningitis, blood is not a good source of viruses.

The India ink preparation is useful for the detection of fungal meningitis such as *Cryptococcus neoformans* (Fig 34). This organism resembles mononuclear cells with Wright's stain (Fig 35) and stains positive with periodic acid-Schiff and methenamine silver stains.

Until quite recently, patients suffering from cryptococcosis were considered to be essentially nonresponsive immunologically. However, various serologic tests that are both diagnostically and prognostically helpful are

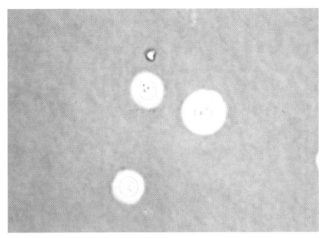

Fig 34. India ink preparation demonstrating *Cryptococcus neoformans*.

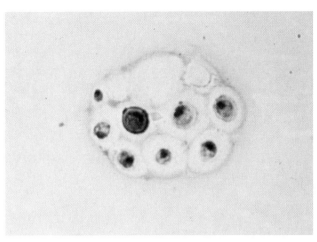

Fig 35. *Cryptococcus neoformans* in a patient being treated for Hodgkin's disease.

now available. These methods include an indirect fluorescent antibody technique, tube agglutination and charcoal particle agglutination for cryptococcal antibodies, and a latex slide agglutination test for cryptococcal antigen. The last test is probably the current procedure of choice, since it is highly specific, has both diagnostic and prognostic value, and is widely used.[81] It can be used with both serum and CSF. False-positive reactions are rare, and the test correlates very well with cultural methods (92% correlation). A positive latex test with CSF at any titer is usually indicative of active CNS disease. The titer is usually proportional to the extent of the infection. Increasing titers suggest spread of the infection and a poor prognosis, while declining titers indicate a good therapeutic response.

In primary amebic meningioencephalitis, organisms such as *Acanthameba* sp and *Nagleria* sp are difficult to identify on stained smears. Wet mount preparations, immunofluorescent methods, and electron microscopy may be helpful in the diagnosis.

Counterimmunoelectrophoresis

The technique of CIE is essentially the familiar Ouchterlony gel-diffusion to which an electric current has been applied. At the pH used (usually 8.6), the water-soluble antigen is strongly negative and migrates toward the anode. The antibody is also negatively charged. Since the antibody charge is so weak, however, it is pulled in a counter direction by the endosmotic forces toward the cathode. The antigen and antibody therefore meet near the center, combine, and precipitate to form a visible band.

The first clinical application of CIE was in 1970 when Gocke and Howe used the method for the identification of the hepatitis B antigen in serum. Shortly thereafter, it was shown to be useful in demonstrating the presence of the antigens of *S pneumoniae* and *N meningitidis*. Improvements in the technique have now made it a reasonably simple, rapid, and reliable method to identify a variety of bacterial antigens and a few antibodies.[82-84] Although applicable to the measurement of all body fluids, including serum and urine, CIE is particularly valuable in cases of suspected bacterial meningitis. Specific bacterial identification can be made within an hour of receiving the spinal fluid. Unfortunately, all microorganisms are not detectable by this technique. Currently, the method is reliable for most types of *S pneumoniae*, *H influenzae*, Group B streptococci, and *N meningitidis*. These organisms, however, are by far the most common ones seen in childhood meningitis, so most infections can be diagnosed by this procedure.

Although the technique is highly specific, it lacks some degree of sensitivity. Occasional cases are seen in which the CIE measurement is negative, but cultures are positive. False-negative values from CIE can be significantly reduced if the CSF is concentrated prior to use. Still, even when this is done, a negative CIE value and positive culture can sometimes occur. In these situations, organisms are invariably rare; and cultures usually show only one to three colonies and require a 36–48-hour incubation period before the organisms are recognized. Analysis of serum and urine by CIE, although positive less often compared to CSF, may also be of assistance in many cases. When CSF, serum, and urine are evaluated simultaneously, the diagnostic accuracy reportedly approaches 100%.[85]

A recent report suggests that an equally accurate diagnosis of bacterial meningitis using latex particle agglutination may soon be possible.[86] This would not only reduce the time needed for analysis but would be much simpler in terms of equipment and technical skills.

Limulus Lysate Gelation Test

The horseshoe crab, *Limulus polyphemus,* is a prehistoric creature mysteriously found only on the eastern coasts of continents. Circulating within it are cells known as amebocytes. These cells contain a copper complex, giving them a blue color. A lysate of the amebocytes has been found to coagulate in the presence of extremely small quantities of endotoxin. This finding led Levin and Bang to develop a relatively simple, rapid, and reliable test that detects endotoxin in various body fluids.[87] It has now been shown to be particularly helpful in the early diagnosis of meningitis due to gram-negative organisms.[88, 89] Its use in the diagnosis of gram-negative sepsis has been less clear-cut and technically more difficult.

The test using CSF is an excellent adjunct to the measurement of lactate and to CIE in the rapid diagnosis of bacterial meningitis. Lactate in the CSF is usually elevated in all types of bacterial meningitis. However, it may also be abnormal in a variety of noninfectious processes. When the results are positive, CIE is highly specific; yet, it lacks sensitivity and is limited to a relatively small group of microorganisms. The Limulus test is positive in essentially all gram-negative infections, including *H influenzae, E coli, N meningitidis, Proteus morganii, Citrobacter freundii,* and *Pseudomonas aeruginosa.* Since wide varieties of gram-negative organisms are known to cause sepsis and meningitis in neonates, the test is particularly helpful in the newborn where rapid diagnosis and treatment are so important.

Since endotoxin is ubiquitous and contamination widespread, adequate precautions must be taken when performing this test.[90]

Tests for Neurosyphilis

The lack of a completely reliable laboratory test for the diagnosis of neurosyphilis means that this diagnosis can be quite difficult to establish and must be based primarily upon clinical findings. This is further complicated by a rising incidence in atypical forms of syphilis, the subtlety of clinical findings, and the fact that nontreponemal serologic tests are not sensitive enough to be of great help in this diagnosis.[91]

Tests for syphilis are basically of two types—those that measure nonspecific antibodies (reagins) and those that measure specific treponemal antibodies. The nonspecific reaginic tests (Serologic Test for Syphilis or STS) include the VDRL, Rapid Plasma Reagin or RPR, Mazzini, and Kolmer tests, among others. The specific tests use a variety of preparations of the treponemal antigen, including *Treponema pallidum* immobilization (TPI), fluorescent treponemal antibody (FTA), fluorescent treponemal antibody with absorption (FTA-ABS), and the microhemagglutination test for *T pallidum* (MHA-TP), among others. The FTA-ABS test has generally replaced the TPI and is considered to be the current standard treponemal test.

The reagin tests, while quite satisfactory for screening patients for syphilis by using serum, lack sensitivity to adequately evaluate the CSF. As a result, at least 40% of the patients with neurosyphilis will have a negative VDRL of the CSF.[92–94] Escobar and associates recommend the highly sensitive FTA test for screening spinal fluid for neurosyphilis. Since this test lacks some specificity, resulting in a few false-positives, the FTA-ABS and VDRL were recommended for all fluids giving a positive FTA. However, a more recent report questions the diagnostic value of the FTA-ABS test with CSF.[95]

In infants with neurosyphilis, the mother will have positive serum VDRL and FTA results in over 90% of the cases. Since these antibodies are primarily IgG, they cross the placenta. Hence, cord bloods will also be positive, regardless of whether the infant has congenital syphilis or not. If available, the specific FTA-ABS-IgM test for specific infant antibodies is very helpful. In any event, the CSF should be examined since asymptomatic neurosyphilis is common in the congenital form of the disease.[94]

References

1. Fishman RA: Cerebrospinal fluid, in Boher AB, Boher LH (eds): Clinical Neurology. New York: Harper & Row, 1971

2. Krieg AF: Cerebrospinal fluids and other body fluids, in Henry JB (ed): Clinical Diagnosis and Management by Laboratory Methods, ed 16. Philadelphia: WB Saunders Co, 1979, pp 635–657

3. Sarff LD, Platt LH, McCracken GH: Cerebrospinal fluid evaluation in neonates: Composition in high-risk infants with and without meningitis. J Pediatr 88:473–477, 1976

4. McCracken GH: Neonatal septicemia and meningitis. Hosp Pract 11:89, 1976

5. Sheth KV: Cerebrospinal and Body Fluids Cell Morphology Through a Hematologist's Microscope, American Society of Clinical Pathologists workshop manual. Chicago: ASCP, 1978

6. Dyken PR: Cerebrospinal fluid cytology: Practical clinical usefulness. Neurology 25:210–217, 1975

7. Kölmel HW: Atlas of Cerebrospinal Fluid Cells, ed 2. New York: Springer-Verlag, 1977

8. Oehmichen M: Cerebrospinal Fluid Cytology. An Introduction and Atlas. Philadelphia: WB Saunders Co, 1976

9. Moser RP, Robinson JA, Prostko ER: Lymphocyte subpopulations in human cerebrospinal fluid. Neurology 26:726–728, 1976

10. Oehmichen M, Huber H: Supplementary cytodiagnostic analysis of mononuclear cells of the cerebrospinal fluid using cytological markers. J Neurol 218:187–196, 1978

11. Traugott U: T and B lymphocytes in the cerebrospinal fluid of various neurological diseases. J Neurol 219:185–197, 1978

12. Bosch I, Oehmichen M: Eosinophilic granulocytes in cerebrospinal fluid: Analysis of 94 cerebrospinal fluid specimens and review of the literature. J Neurol 219:93–105, 1978

13. Kuberski T: Eosinophils in the cerebrospinal fluid. Ann Intern Med 91:70–75, 1979

14. Glasser L, Corrigan JJ, Payne C: Basophilic meningitis secondary to lymphoma. Neurology 26:899–902, 1976

15. Nosanchuk JS, Kim CW: Lupus erythematosus cells in CSF. JAMA 25:2,883–2,884, 1976

16. Balhuizen JC, et al: Value of cerebrospinal fluid cytology for the diagnosis of malignancies in the central nervous system. J Neurosurg 48:747–753, 1978

17. Gondos B: Cytology of cerebrospinal fluid: Technical and diagnostic considerations. Ann Clin Lab Sci 6:152–157, 1976

18. Chartrand SA, Cho CT: Persistent pleocytosis in bacterial meningitis. J Pediatr 88:424–426, 1976

19. Aaronson AG, Hajdu SI, Melamed MR: Spinal fluid cytology during chemotherapy of leukemia of the central nervous system in children. Am J Clin Pathol 63:523–537, 1975

20. Ducos R, et al: Sedimentation versus cytocentrifugation in the cytologic study of craniospinal fluid. Cancer 43:479–482, 1979

21. Drewinko B, Sullivan MP, Martin T: Use of the cytocentrifuge in the diagnosis of meningeal leukemia. Cancer 31:1,331–1,336, 1973

22. Gondos B, King EG: Cerebrospinal fluid cytology: Diagnostic accuracy and comparison of different techniques. Acta Cytol 21:542–547, 1976

23. Bunn PA, et al: Central nervous system complications in patients with diffuse histiocytic and undifferentiated lymphoma: Leukemia revisited. Blood 47:3–10, 1976

24. Young RC, et al: Central nervous system complications of non-Hodgkin's lymphomas. Am J Med 66:435–443, 1979

25. Tibbling G, Link H, Ohma S: Principles of albumin and IgG analysis in neurological disorders. I. Establishment of reference values. Scand J Clin Lab Invest 37:385–390, 1977

26. Schriever H, Gambino S: Protein turbidity produced by trichloroacetic acid and sulfosalicylic acid at varying temperatures and varying ratios of albumin and globulin. Am J Clin Pathol 44:667–672, 1975

27. Lowry OH, et al: Protein measurement with the Folin-phenol reagent. J Biol Chem 193:265–275, 1951

28. Patrick RL, Thiers RE: The direct spectrophotometric determination of protein in cerebrospinal fluid. Clin Chem 9:283–295, 1963

29. Igou PC: An evaluation of a gel filtration-spectrophotometric method for spinal fluid protein. Am J Med Technol 33:354–360, 1967

30. Pesce MA, Strande CS: A new micromethod for determination of protein in cerebrospinal fluid and urine. Clin Chem 19:1,265–1,267, 1973

31. Kaplan A: Electrophoresis of cerebrospinal fluid proteins. Am J Med Sci 253:549–555, 1967

32. Windisch RM, Bracken MM: Cerebrospinal fluid proteins: Concentration by membrane ultrafiltration and fractionation by electrophoresis on cellulose acetate. Clin Chem 16:416–419, 1970

33. Breebaart L, Becker H, Jongebloed FA: Investigation of reference values of components of cerebrospinal fluid. J Clin Chem Clin Biochem 16:561–565, 1978

34. Ivers RR, et al: Spinal-fluid gamma globulin in multiple sclerosis and other neurologic diseases. JAMA 176:515–519, 1961

35. Link H, Muller R: Immunoglobulins in multiple sclerosis and infections of the nervous system. Arch Neurol 25:326–344, 1971

36. Johnson KP, et al: Agarose electrophoresis of cerebrospinal fluid in multiple sclerosis. Neurology 27:273–277, 1977

37. Tourtellotte WW, et al: Cerebrospinal fluid electroimmunodiffusion. Arch Neurol 25:345–350, 1971

38. Kabat EA, Moore DH, Landow H: An electrophoretic study of the protein component in cerebrospinal fluid and their relationship to the serum proteins. J Clin Invest 21:571–577, 1942

39. Kabat EA, Glusman M, Knaub V: Quantitative estimation of the albumin and gamma globulin in normal and pathologic cerebrospinal fluid by immunochemical methods. Am J Med 4:653–662, 1948

40. Hartley TF, Merrill DA, Claman HN: Quantitation of immunoglobulins in cerebrospinal fluid. Arch Neurol 15:472–479, 1966

41. Joseph JC, Bermes EW: Comparison of protein values in cerebrospinal fluid by nephelometry and radial immunodiffusion. Ann Clin Lab Sci 9:408–415, 1979

42. Link H, Zetterwall O: Multiple sclerosis: disturbed kappa:lambda light chain ratio of immunoglobulin G in cerebrospinal fluid. Clin Exp Immunol 6:435–438, 1970

43. Palmer DL, Minard BJ, Witt NJ: IgG subgroups of multiple sclerosis dysproteins. Am J Clin Pathol 59:140, 1973

44. Cohen SR, Herndon RM, McKhann GM: Radioimmunoassay of myelin basic protein in spinal fluid. N Engl J Med 295:1,455–1,457, 1976

45. Menkes JH: The causes for low spinal fluid sugar in bacterial meningitis: Another look. Pediatrics 44:1–3, 1969

46. Swartz MN, Dodge PR: Bacterial meningitis—A review of selected aspects. N Engl J Med 272:779–787, 1965

47. Feldman WE: Cerebrospinal fluid lactic acid dehydrogenase activity. Levels in untreated and partially antibiotic-treated meningitis. Am J Dis Child 129:77–80, 1975

48. Controni G, et al: Cerebrospinal fluid lactic acid levels in meningitis. J Pediatr 92:379–384, 1977

49. Hull HF, Morrow G: Glucorrhea revisited. Prolonged promulgation of another plastic pearl. JAMA 234:1,052–1,053, 1975

50. Savory J, Brody JP: Measurement and diagnostic value of cerebrospinal fluid enzymes. Ann Clin Lab Sci 9:68–79, 1979

51. Wroblewski F, Decker B, Wroblewski R: The clinical implications of spinal-fluid lactic dehydrogenase activity. N Engl J Med 258:635–639, 1958

52. Feldman WE: Cerebrospinal fluid lactic acid dehydrogenase activity. Levels in untreated and partially antibiotic-treated meningitis. Am J Dis Child 129:77–80, 1975

53. Nelson PV, Carney WF, Pollard AC: Diagnostic significance and source of lactate dehydrogenase and its isoenzymes in cerebrospinal fluid of children with a variety of neurological disorders. J Clin Pathol 28:828–833, 1975

54. Beaty HN, Oppenheimer S: Cerebrospinal-fluid lactic dehydrogenase and its isoenzymes in infections of the central nervous system. N Engl J Med 279:1,197–1,202, 1968

55. Florez G, et al: Changes in serum and cerebrospinal fluid enzyme activity after head injury. Acta Neurochir 35:3–13, 1976

56. Rabe EF, Curnen EC: The occurrence of lysozyme in the cerebrospinal fluid and serum of infants and children. Pediatrics 38:147–153, 1951

57. Di Lorenzo N, Palma L, Ferrante L: Cerebrospinal fluid lysozyme activity in patients with central nervous system tumors. Neurochirurgia 20:19–22, 1977

58. Jaikin A, Agrust A: Cerebrospinal fluid glutamine concentration in patients with chronic hypercapnea. Clin Sci 36:11–14, 1969

59. Glasgow AM, Dhiensiri K: Improved assay for spinal fluid glutamine, and values for children with Reye's syndrome. Clin Chem 29:642–644, 1974

60. Whitehead TP, Whittaker SRF: A method for the determination of glutamine in cerebrospinal fluid and the results in hepatic coma. J Clin Pathol 8:81–84, 1955

61. Hourani BT, Hamlin EM, Reynolds TB: Cerebrospinal fluid glutamine as a measure of hepatic encephalopathy. Arch Intern Med 127:1,033–1,036, 1971

62. Moir ATB, et al: Cerebral metabolites in cerebrospinal fluid as a biochemical approach to the brain. Brain 93:357–368, 1970

63. Jakupcevic M, et al: Nonhomogeneous distribution of 5-hydroxyindoleacetic acid and homovanillic acid in the lumbar cerebrospinal fluid of man. J Neurol Sci 31:165–171, 1977

64. Waterbury LD, Pearce LA: Separation and identification of neutral and acidic metabolites in cerebrospinal fluid. Clin Chem 18:258–262, 1972

65. Perry TL, Hansen S, Christie RG: Amino compounds and organic acids in CSF, plasma, and urine of autistic children. Biol Psychiatry 13:575–586, 1978

66. Perry TL, et al: Nonketotic hyperglycinemia: Glycine accumulation due to absence of glycine cleavage in brain. N Engl J Med 292:1,269–1,273, 1975

67. Sjaastad O, et al: Homocarnosinosis. 2. A familial metabolic disorder associated with spastic paraplegia, pro-

gressive mental deficiency and retinal pigmentation. Acta Neurol Scand 53:275–290, 1976

68. Sambrook MA: The concentration of cerebrospinal fluid potassium during systemic disturbances of acid-base metabolism. J Clin Pathol 28:418–420, 1975
69. Siemkowicz E, Christiansen I, Sorensen S: Changes in cisternal fluid potassium concentration following cardiac arrest. Acta Neurol Scand 55:137–144, 1977
70. Woodbury J, et al: Cerebrospinal fluid and serum levels of magnesium, zinc, and calcium in man. Neurology 18:700–705, 1965
71. Levinson A: The hydrogen-ion concentration of cerebrospinal fluid: Studies in meningitis. J Inf Dis 21:556–570, 1917
72. Bland RD, Lister RC, Ries JP: Cerebrospinal fluid lactic acid level and pH in meningitis. Am J Dis Child 128:151–156, 1974
73. Wichser J, Kazemi H: CSF bicarbonate regulation in respiratory acidosis and alkalosis. J Appl Physiol 38:504–512, 1975
74. Plum F, Siesjo BK: Recent advances in CSF physiology. Anesthesiology 42:708–730, 1975
75. Katsurada K, et al: Cerebrospinal fluid acidosis and its possible relation to acute brain swelling. Jpn J Surg 2:131–140, 1972
76. Pryce JD, Gant PW, Saul KJ: Normal concentrations of lactate, glucose and protein in cerebrospinal fluid, and the diagnostic implications of abnormal concentrations. Clin Chem 16:562–565, 1970
77. Bland RD, Lister RC, Ries JP: CSF lactic acid levels and pH in meningitis. Am J Dis Child 128:151–156, 1974
78. Controni G, et al: Cerebrospinal fluid lactic acid levels in meningitis. J Pediatr 92:379–384, 1977
79. Brook I, et al: Measurement of lactic acid in cerebrospinal fluid of patients with infections of central nervous system. J Infect Dis 137:384–390, 1978
80. Knight JA, Dudek SM, Haymond RE: Increased cerebrospinal fluid lactate and early diagnosis of bacterial meningitis. Clin Chem 25:809–810, 1979
81. Kaufman L: Serodiagnosis of fungal diseases, in Rose NR, Friedman H (eds): Manual of Clinical Immunology. Washington, DC: American Society for Microbiology, 1976, pp 371–372
82. Dorff GJ, Coonrod JD, Rytel MW: Detection by immunoelectrophoresis of antigen in sera of patients with pneumococcal bacteremia. Lancet 1:578–579, 1971
83. Edwards EA, Muehl PM, Peckinpaugh RO: Diagnosis of bacterial meningitis by counterimmunoelectrophoresis. J Lab Clin Med 80:449–454, 1972
84. Rytel MW: Counterimmunoelectrophoresis in diagnosis of infectious disease. Hosp Pract 10:75–82, 1975
85. Feigin RD, et al: Countercurrent immunoelectrophoresis of urine as well as of CSF and blood for diagnosis of bacterial meningitis. J Pediatr 89:773–775, 1976
86. Ward JI, et al: Rapid diagnosis of *Hemophilus influenzae* type B infections by latex particle agglutination and counterimmunoelectrophoresis. J Pediatr 93:37–42, 1978
87. Levin J, Bang FB: Clotable protein in limulus. Its localization and kinetics of its coagulation by endotoxin. Thromb Diath Haemorrh 19:186–197, 1968
88. Nachum R, Lipsfy A, Siegel SE: Rapid detection of gram-negative bacterial meningitis by the limulus lysate test. N Engl J Med 289:931–934, 1973
89. Dyson D, Cassaday G: Use of limulus lysate for detecting gram-negative neonatal meningitis. Pediatrics 58:105–109, 1976
90. Riegle L, Cooperstock MS: Limulus gelation test: Laboratory considerations. Lab Med 8:28–30, 1977
91. Hooshmand H, Escobar MR, Kopf SW: Neurosyphilis. JAMA 219:726–729, 1972
92. Harner RE, Smith JL, Israel CW: The FTA-ABS test in late syphilis: A serological study in 1,985 cases. JAMA 293:545–548, 1968
93. Escobar MR, Dalton HP, Allison MJ: Fluorescent antibody tests for syphilis using cerebrospinal fluid: Clinical correlation in 150 cases. Am J Clin Pathol 53:886–890, 1970
94. McCracken GH, Kaplan JM: Penicillin treatment for congenital syphilis: A critical reappraisal. JAMA 228:855–858, 1974
95. Lee TJ, Sparling PF: Syphilis: An algorithm. JAMA 242:1,187–1,189, 1979

2 Pleural and Pericardial Fluids

Anatomy and Physiology

The pleura encloses the lungs and consists of a thin membrane that forms a double layer. The two layers are contiguous, and the space between them forms the *pleural cavity,* which is lined by a single layer of mesothelial cells (the mesothelium). Normally, the two layers of mesothelium are separated only by small amounts of fluid that facilitate movement of the two membranes against each other. The pleural cavity is, therefore, not a true cavity but only becomes so in the presence of disease causing the accumulation of fluid therein.

Similarly, the *pericardial cavity* is only a potential cavity formed by two serous membranes that are closely apposed to each other and separated by small amounts of serous fluid. This fluid allows the heart to move easily during contraction and relaxation. Following injury or the onset of disease, fluid may accumulate within the cavity, causing a separation between the visceral and parietal pericardia.

The accumulation of fluid within the pleural or pericardial cavities is called an *effusion.*

Pleural fluid is being formed and absorbed constantly. This fluid is formed by the filtration of plasma through capillary endothelium. Its presence is dependent on the hydrostatic pressure in capillaries, plasma osmotic pressure, lymphatic resorption, and permea-bility of capillaries.[1,2] Fluid is reabsorbed by lymphatics and venules in the pleura.

Accumulation of pleural fluid (pleural effusion) may result from increased hydrostatic pressure in the systemic circulation, decreased plasma osmotic pressure, increased permeability of the capillaries in the pleura, and decreased lymphatic resorption. The presence of approximately 300 ml of pleural fluid is required before it can be detected by a chest X-ray. Causes of pleural effusions are listed in Table 2-1. Pleural transudates, which are frequently bilateral and due to hydrodynamic imbalance, are usually diagnosed easily as being due to congestive heart failure, nephrotic syndrome, cirrhosis, or malnutrition. The pathogenesis of exudative effusions may be more difficult to diagnose. Pleural effusions often develop during the course of bacterial pneumonia and usually resolve spontaneously.

Unilateral pleural effusion, particularly on the right side, may result from disease below the diaphragm such as a subdiaphragmatic abscess, hepatic abscess, acute pancreatitis, and tumors. Pleural effusions are common in systemic lupus erythematosus (SLE) but may be due to congestive heart failure or nephrotic syndrome. Rheumatoid arthritis may be associated with an inflammatory pleural reaction. Pleural effusions are common in the first few days after abdominal surgery

Table 2–1. Causes of Pleural Effusion*

Transudates
Congestive heart failure
Cirrhosis
Hypoproteinemia (nephrotic syndrome)

Exudates
Infections
Neoplasms
Pulmonary infarction
Trauma
Pancreatitis
Rheumatoid arthritis
Systemic lupus erythematosus

Chylous Effusion
Trauma
Lymphoma
Carcinoma
Tuberculosis

*Adapted from Krieg.[3] Used by permission.

but usually resolve spontaneously. In the majority of cases they are associated with atelectasis, peritoneal fluid, or irritation of the diaphragm.[4]

Accumulation of fluid in the pericardial cavity (pericardial effusion) is most frequently caused by damage to the lining of the pericardial cavity with an increase in capillary permeability. Disorders associated with pericardial effusion are listed in Table 2–2.

Transudates and Exudates

Effusions of pleural, pericardial, or peritoneal cavities may be divided into transudates and exudates. In general, transudates indicate that fluid has accumulated due to a systemic disease. A common disorder associated with transudates is congestive heart failure. Exudates are usually associated with disorders involving the pleural surfaces such as inflammation, malignancy, or infection (see Table 2–1).

Table 2–2. Causes of Pericardial Effusion*

Exudates
Infections
Myocardial infarction
Neoplasms
Trauma
Uremia

*Adapted from Krieg.[3] Used by permission.

Many criteria are used to separate transudates from exudates; but none of these are absolutely reliable, and there may be considerable overlap among them. The most useful laboratory criteria for identifying exudative pleural fluids are (1) total protein greater than 3 gm/dl, (2) pleural fluid lactate dehydrogenase (LD) content of 200 IU or more, (3) a ratio of pleural fluid to serum LD of 0.6 or more, and (4) a pleural fluid RBC count of 100,000 cells/μl or more.[5] The laboratory criteria for separating transudates and exudates in pericardial fluid are not well defined. This is, however, usually not important since most clinically significant pericardial effusions are exudates.

The most important elements in the diagnostic approach to any effusion are a careful history and physical examination of the patient. Pleural effusion may be caused by diseases of the pleura or of another intrathoracic organ, and abdominal or systemic disorders. To properly manage a pleural or pericardial effusion, the exact diagnosis of the underlying disease must be determined. Aspiration of a significant effusion is frequently indicated, and appropriate laboratory examination of the fluid often gives an important clue to the diagnosis.

Gross Examination

The first step in the investigation of pleural and pericardial effusions is the gross examination, which can play an important role in determining the pathogenesis of the effusion.[3, 6] Massive pleural effusions that occupy the entire hemithorax are most commonly associated with malignancy.[7] The most common type of malignancy associated with massive pleural effusions is carcinoma of the lung followed by breast carcinoma. Cirrhosis of the liver and congestive heart failure may also be associated with massive effusions.

Transudates are usually clear, pale yellow, and do not clot. *Exudates* are cloudy to purulent, and often clot while standing due to the presence of fibrinogen. The latter fluid is usually associated with large numbers of leukocytes and an elevated protein content. The presence of clearly visible pus is diagnostic of empyema.

Hemorrhagic fluid may be due to a traumatic tap, malignancy, pulmonary infarction, trauma, pancreatitis, or tuberculosis. It should be noted that it takes only 2 ml of peripheral blood in 1,000 ml of pleural fluid to produce a blood-tinged appearance.[8] A traumatic tap must be distinguished from other causes of blood in the pleural fluid. In a traumatic tap, the blood is usually nonuniform in distribution and gradually clears as aspiration proceeds. The most common cause of hemorrhagic effusions is malignancy (usually lung cancer). True hemothorax, as may be seen in chest injuries, is associated with pure blood in the pleural cavity. A hematocrit may be used for differentiating true hemothorax from hemorrhagic effusions. In a true hemothorax, the hematocrit of the fluid will be similar to that of the peripheral blood.

Chylous or so-called *pseudochylous effusions* are typified by milky-white pleural fluids. A true chylothorax is rare and is due to the leakage of thoracic ducts, usually caused by trauma or malignancy.[9] In rare cases, it may be the presenting sign of a lymphoma. Pseudochylous fluid, which may be due to chronic effusions from such causes as rheumatoid arthritis or tuberculosis, has a milky or greenish appearance, and sometimes has a silky sheen. This appearance is due to cellular debris and cholesterol crystals.

True chylous fluid clears and decreases in volume with alkalinization or extraction with ether after acidification with hydrochloric acid.[3] Fat droplets, which may be seen with polarized light and by staining with Sudan III, can be demonstrated in chylous fluid. Lipoprotein electrophoresis of chylous fluid shows markedly elevated chylomicrons that are usually scanty or absent in pseudochylous effusions.[10] In pseudochylous effusions, the cholesterol level is usually greater than 145 mg/dl, and cholesterol crystals can be demonstrated with microscopic examination. The differentiation of chylous from pseudochylous effusion may also be made following ingestion of lipophilic dye and with a lymphangiogram. The dye will appear in true chylous effusions after 12–24 hours but will not be seen in pseudochylous effusions.[3]

Cell Counts

Total leukocyte counts are of limited value in the differential diagnosis of pleural and pericardial effusions.[11] In general, leukocyte counts less than 1,000/μl are associated with transudates, while leukocyte counts greater than 1,000/μl are seen in exudates. These values should not, however, be relied on to separate exudates from transudates, since there is considerable overlap.

The usefulness of the RBC count is also limited. This may be related to the fact that it takes so little peripheral blood to give a red appearance to the serous fluid.

However, RBC counts greater than 10,000/μl are highly suggestive of malignant neoplasm, trauma, or pulmonary infarction.

Microscopic Examination

An examination of the cells present and a differential count should be performed on a stained smear made by using cytocentrifugation, Millipore* filtration, or sedimentation methods. The cell types encountered in pleural, pericardial, and peritoneal fluids are neutrophils (PMNs, eosinophils, and basophils); lymphocytes; plasma cells; mononuclear phagocytes (monocytes, histiocytes, and macrophages); mesothelial cells; and malignant cells. The following description refers to these cells seen in pleural, pericardial, and peritoneal fluids.

Mesothelial cells, which form the lining of pleural, pericardial, and peritoneal cavities, usually cause the most difficulty during the evaluation of the cell types present (Fig 36). During inflammatory processes, mesothelial cells undergo proliferation and often desquamate into the serous fluid. They may appear singly or in clusters (Fig 37). The cells are large and measure 12–30 μ in diameter. The cytoplasm is abundant, light grey to deep blue, and may have a perinuclear zone of pallor, giving a "fried egg" appearance (Fig 38). Small cytoplasmic vacuoles may be seen. The nucleus is round to oval and occupies about one third to one half of the cell's diameter. The chromatin is stippled and dark purple (Fig 39). One to three nucleoli may be seen. This description refers to the appearance of mesothelial cells treated with Wright's or May-Grünwald stain.

The mesothelial cells vary in appearance and often show atypical or so-called reactive changes. They are commonly mistaken for malignant cells. Mesothelial cells may be multinucleated, occasionally containing 20 or more nuclei; sometimes clusters or sheets of cells are seen (Figs 40–42). Clusters may be caused by centrifugation, and in cases of long-standing effusion, may closely resemble malignant cells (Fig 43). Clumps of mesothelial cells may be differentiated from malignant cells by comparing the appearance of the mesothelial cells within a clump with other, more readily identifiable mesothelial cells in the same smear, thereby recognizing the "family similarity." The uni-

---

*Millipore Corporation, Bedford, MA 01730.

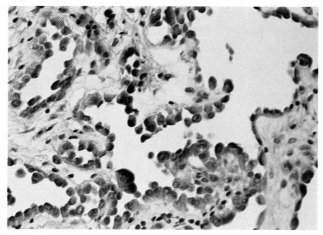

Fig 36. A section of pleura showing lining of mesothelial cells (H & E stain).

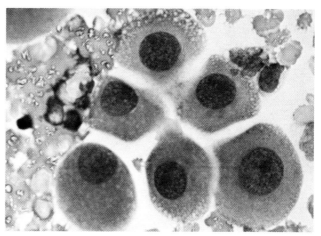

Fig 39. Mesothelial cells with stippled, dark purple chromatin.

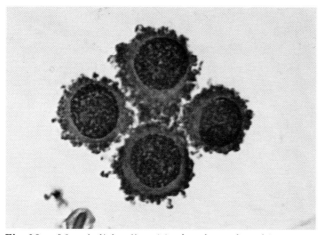

Fig 37. Mesothelial cells in pleural fluid.

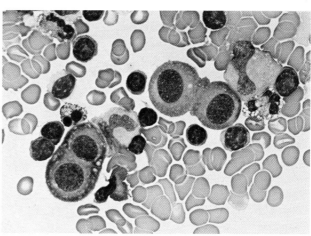

Fig 40. Binucleated mesothelial cells and lymphocytes in peritoneal fluid.

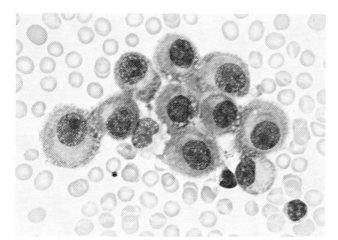

Fig 38. Mesothelial cells with abundant, deep blue cytoplasm and a paranuclear halo in pleural fluid.

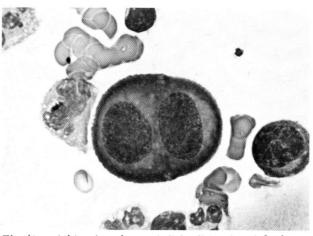

Fig 41. A binucleated mesothelial cell in pleural fluid.

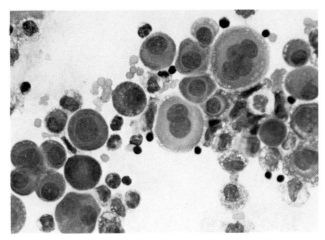

Fig 42. Mesothelial cells of varying sizes, including multinucleated forms found in pleural fluid.

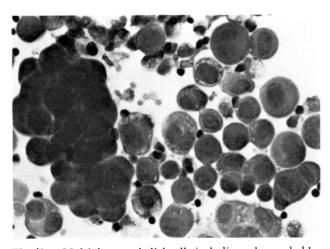

Fig 43. Multiple mesothelial cells including a large, darkly stained cluster that could be mistaken for malignant cells in pleural fluid.

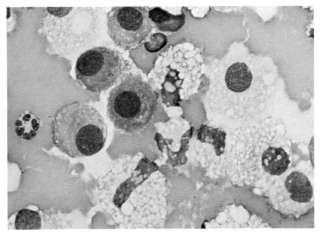

Fig 44. Mesothelial cells resembling plasma cells and macrophages in pleural fluid.

form, regular arrangement of the cells indicates their benign origin.

Degenerative mesothelial cells may show pyknosis and karyorrhexis, and occasionally resemble plasma cells (Fig 44). Mesothelial cells may exhibit phagocytosis and transformation into macrophages.[12] It may, therefore, be extremely difficult to differentiate mononuclear phagocytes from intermediate forms of mesothelial cells. The nonspecific esterase stain is not useful in differentiating mesothelial cells, mononuclear phagocytes, and malignant cells from one another, since strong enzyme activity may be present in all of these cells.[12, 13]

Mesothelial cells are seen in variable numbers in most effusions and are increased in sterile inflammations caused by conditions such as pneumonia, pulmonary infarction, and malignancy. In tuberculous pleurisy or when heavy concentrations of pyogenic organisms are present within the serous cavities, mesothelial cells are usually scarce.[14] This is probably due to a fibrinous exudate covering the mesothelial lining of the cavity.

Neutrophils (PMNs) differ in appearance in serous fluids. They may appear more or less identical to those seen in the blood (Fig 45) or may be difficult to recognize as being PMNs.[14] In long-standing effusions, the granules may be decreased or lost. The nuclei may appear as densely stained, spherical fragments and are sometimes mistaken for nucleated RBCs (Fig 46). Occasionally, the cytoplasm may have a bluish color so that the PMN may resemble a lymphocyte. In infected effusions, PMNs may show evidence of degeneration in the form of vacuolation, loss of granules, and blurred nuclei.

It is debatable how valuable a differential leukocyte count is in the differential diagnosis. The number of PMNs present in all effusions may vary, but a predominance of PMNs suggests bacterial pneumonia, pulmonary infarction, or pancreatitis. Serous fluid neutrophilia is usually the initial cellular reaction to these conditions. Later, there may be a predominance of mononuclear cells and mesothelial cells.

Lymphocytes are seen in variable numbers in most serous effusions (Figs 47 and 48). They may be small, medium, or large; and they may exhibit reactive changes. The lymphocytes may have an immature appearance, suggesting lymphocytic leukemia or lymphoma if they represent the predominant cell type. Nucleoli are often more prominent than in the peripheral blood lymphocytes (Fig 49), and the nuclei may be

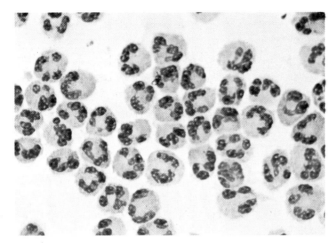

Fig 45. Neutrophilic reaction in a patient with acute peritonitis.

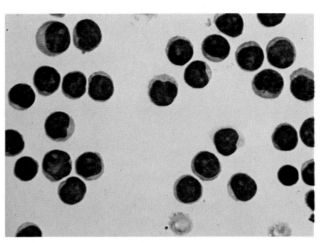

Fig 48. Lymphocytosis of the pleural fluid in a patient with tuberculosis. Note that mesothelial cells are not present.

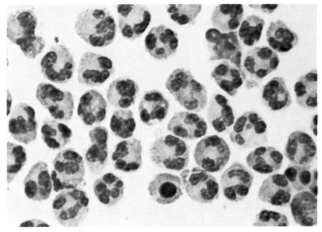

Fig 46. Neutrophilic reaction including a neutrophil with a pyknotic nucleus, simulating a nucleated RBC from the pleural fluid of a patient with bacterial pneumonia.

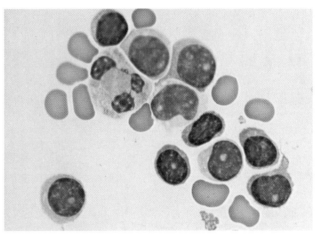

Fig 49. Lymphocytes with prominent nucleoli in a patient with nephrotic syndrome.

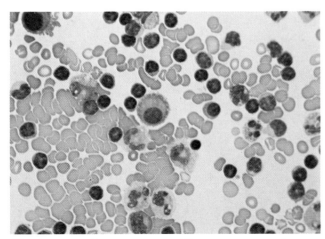

Fig 47. Lymphocytes, neutrophils, monocytes, and a mesothelial cell from the pleural fluid of a patient with congestive heart failure.

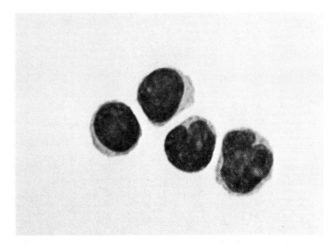

Fig 50. Lymphocytes in peritoneal fluid, two of which have clefted nuclei.

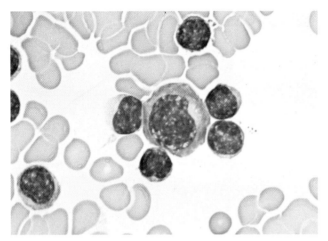

Fig 51. A large atypical, reactive, or transformed lymphocyte, surrounded by smaller lymphocytes in pleural fluid.

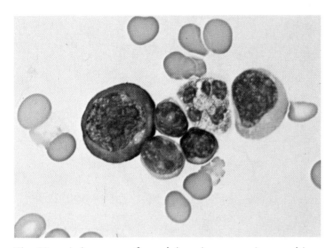

Fig 52. A large transformed lymphocyte or immunoblast with basophilic cytoplasm, surrounded by smaller lymphocytes.

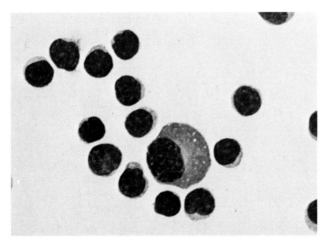

Fig 53. Lymphocytes and a plasma cell in the pleural fluid of a patient with rheumatoid arthritis.

clefted (Fig 50). Some of the irregularity of the nuclear contours may be caused by centrifugation during the concentration process. Transformed or reactive lymphocytes (immunoblasts) may be present (Figs 51 and 52). These are large lymphocytes with abundant deep-blue cytoplasm, and often several prominent nucleoli are evident. Tuberculous and malignant effusions frequently show a predominance of lymphocytes (see Fig 48).[8] In tuberculosis, the fluid characteristically shows lymphocytosis and only a few mesothelial cells. It should be emphasized, however, that the absence of lymphocytosis does not rule out either tuberculosis or malignant effusions. In non-Hodgkin's lymphoma, the malignant lymphocytes are generally uniform in size, shape, and staining characteristics. This is in contrast to a benign condition where there is usually a mixture of different types of lymphocytes. Lymphocytic pleural effusions may also be associated with leakage of the thoracic duct. A lesser degree of lymphocytosis may be seen in congestive heart failure and cirrhosis.

The determination of T- and B-lymphocytes in pleural effusions may aid in the differential diagnosis. In pulmonary tuberculosis, the number of T-lymphocytes in pleural fluid has been reported to be considerably higher than in the peripheral blood.[15] The number of B-lymphocytes in pleural fluid is said to be significantly lower than in peripheral blood from patients with pulmonary tuberculosis, pulmonary malignancy, or nonspecific pleuritis.[15] The presence of a monoclonal B-cell population is suggestive of a malignant lymphoma.

Plasma cells may be seen in fluids from patients with rheumatoid arthritis, malignancy, tuberculosis, and other conditions associated with lymphocytosis (Fig 53).

Pleural fluid *eosinophilia,* like blood eosinophilia, is nonspecific, and it has been described in a number of disorders including infections, pneumothorax, neoplasms, infarction, chest trauma, subdiaphragmatic inflammation, congestive heart failure, collagen diseases, and hypersensitivity states (Fig 54).[16] The pleural fluid eosinophilia may or may not be accompanied by blood eosinophilia. When blood eosinophilia is present, one should consider the possibility of hydatid disease, Löffler's syndrome, periarteritis nodosa, trauma, or Hodgkin's disease. Eosinophilic pleural effusions are usually unilateral and frequently blood-tinged.[16]

Mononuclear phagocytes (monocytes, histiocytes, and macrophages) are usually seen in variable numbers in pleural, pericardial, and peritoneal effusions.[14] Since both monocytes and mesothelial cells may transform into macrophages, the distinction between them is not always obvious (Fig 55). The terms, "macrophage" and "histiocyte," are used synonymously in this book, although some authors distinguish between the two by insisting that the macrophage show evidence of phagocytosis. The macrophages vary in size and have a diameter of 15–25 μ. The cytoplasm is pale grey, cloudy, and frequently vacuolated (Fig 56). Sometimes, very large (up to 50 μ) macrophages may be seen. So-called signet-ring cells are formed when the small vacuoles fuse, forming one or two large ones that flatten the nucleus against the side of the cell membrane (Fig 57). The "signet-ring" cell is a descriptive term and may be seen equally in benign and malignant cells. Macrophages may contain phagocytosed RBCs, hemosiderin (brown or blue particles), portions of PMNs, carbon particles, or yellow bile pigment (Fig 58). Their numbers vary in both benign and malignant fluids and usually increase as the process becomes chronic.

In vivo, *lupus erythematosus (LE)* cell formation has been documented in pleural, pericardial, and peritoneal fluids (Fig 59).[17] However, this finding is rare.

Clinical Correlations

Pleural effusions are found in approximately 50% of the patients with pulmonary embolism.[18] Unfortunately, the fluid usually reveals no diagnostic features. The results of both the gross and microscopic examinations are variable. In more than half of the effusions, the fluid is bloody and initially shows a predominance of PMNs. Later, lymphocytes and macrophages predominate. However, less than two thirds of the fluids tested in one study were exudates. Thus, the presence of clear pleural fluid does not exclude the possibility of pulmonary embolism.[18]

Bacterial pericarditis is characterized by leukocytosis (>1,000/μl) with a predominance of PMNs. Similar findings may be observed in viral pericarditis and postmyocardial infarction syndrome.

Pleural and pericardial effusions have been reported in *uremia* and in patients undergoing *chronic dialysis*.[19, 20] The pleural effusion is usually unilateral, serosanguineous or hemorrhagic, and contains a predominance of lymphocytes. The fluid is usually an exudate. Creatinine levels are similar to those in the blood.

Neoplastic disease is one of the most common causes of

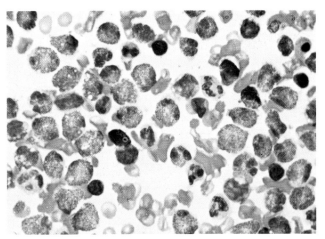

Fig 54. Pleural fluid eosinophilia in a patient with traumatic chest injuries.

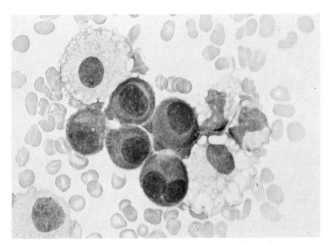

Fig 55. Mixture of mesothelial cells with deep blue cytoplasm and macrophages with multiple phagocytic vacuoles and pale cytoplasm.

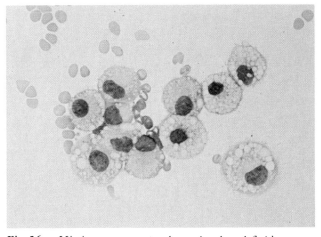

Fig 56. Histiocytes or macrophages in pleural fluid.

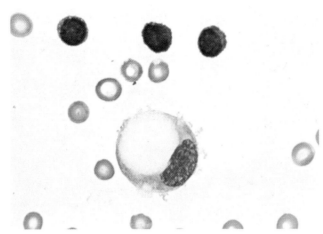

Fig 57. "Signet ring" type macrophage in pleural fluid.

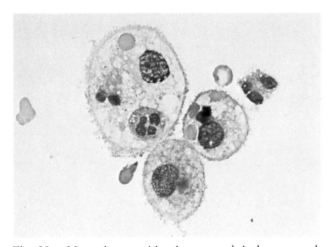

Fig 58. Macrophages with phagocytosed leukocytes and RBCs in pleural fluid.

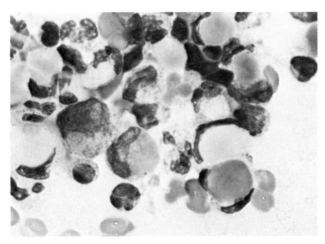

Fig 59. Pleural fluid containing LE cells.

pleural and pericardial effusions.[21, 22] Therefore, the most important part of the laboratory investigation is the examination of smears for malignant cells. Pleural effusions develop in nearly half of the patients with disseminated lung and breast cancer. Effusions are also common in patients with lymphoma,[23] mesothelioma, various sarcomas, and ovarian and gastrointestinal neoplasms. A true chylous effusion is often associated with lymphoma.[24] Carcinoma or lymphoma is the most likely cause of bilateral effusion in the absence of congestive heart failure.

Malignant neoplasms produce pleural effusions through a number of different mechanisms.[21] The neoplasm may produce lymphatic and capillary obstruction, resulting in reduced absorption of fluid and protein. In addition, malignant cells may produce chemical mediators that increase capillary permeability. Neoplastic lesions may also lead to airway obstruction, secondary infection, and local inflammation. Occasionally, the tumor erodes into a blood vessel causing hemothorax.

Malignant effusions are usually exudates. The leukocyte count is variable and may show a predominance of lymphocytes, although serous fluid neutrophilia may also be present. The number of malignant cells found in effusions associated with malignant neoplasms varies.[21] Bilateral effusions are often associated with obstruction of the lymphatics. When this occurs, a cytologic study of the effusion often reveals no malignant cells. In contrast, many malignant cells may be seen where there are free-growing tumor cells within the fluid and in the adjacent pleura. Exfoliation of solid tumor implants in the pleura is associated with a moderate number of tumor cells.

When malignancy is suspected, a specimen should be sent to the cytology laboratory. The smear, prepared as part of the routine examination of the pleural fluid in the clinical laboratory, should also be carefully examined for possible malignant cells. In general, the more methods that are employed to detect possible malignant cells, the better the chance of arriving at a correct diagnosis. No single microscopic feature is absolutely diagnostic of malignant cells, but several points are helpful. Tumor cells frequently aggregate in clumps or cell balls and sometimes show gland-like formation (Fig 60). These clumps of cells are frequently best seen when scanning the smear under low power. Malignant cells usually look distinctly different from cells normally encountered in benign fluids. They often have large nuclei with prominent, abnormally shaped nucleoli. The nuclear to cytoplasmic ratio is usually increased.[14]

Most malignant effusions are caused by metastatic adenocarcinoma. These tumors may be associated with multiple, round, cell aggregates with or without giant vacuoles; or the tumor cells may be isolated and have bizarre, monstrous forms (Fig 61). Atypical mesothelial cells may be difficult to differentiate from malignant cells, as aforementioned. Transmission- and scanning electron-microscopic techniques are occasionally helpful in distinguishing between atypical mesothelial cells and malignant cells.[25, 26]

Oat cell carcinoma of the lung has a very characteristic cell morphology. These cells resemble large lymphocytes but are larger (about 20 μ). The nuclear chromatin is less fine than found in lymphoblasts, and the nucleoli are usually indistinct. The cytoplasmic borders are indistinct, and the cells are often seen in small groups with the nuclei showing "molding" or a mosaic pattern (Fig 62).

Malignant pleural effusions are associated with metastatic breast carcinoma (Fig 63), mesothelioma (Fig 64), malignant lymphoma (Figs 65 and 66), and leukemia (Fig 67). Lymphomatoid granulomatosis is associated with a variety of bizarre lymphoid cells and may be difficult to differentiate from a malignant lymphoma (Fig 68).

In addition to the examination of the pleural fluid, a *needle biopsy* of the pleura may significantly enhance the diagnostic yield.[27, 28] This is readily performed at the time of the initial thoracentesis or later, depending on the clinical situation and the laboratory results. A closed pleural biopsy should be performed on all undiagnosed exudates. An open thoracotomy or fiber-optic pleuroscopy may be useful for a definitive diagnosis. A pleural biopsy is particularly useful for the diagnosis of malignancy and tuberculosis. If the latter is suspected, a portion of the biopsy should be submitted for culture.

Metastatic tumors to the pericardium and the heart are common in patients with advanced malignant disease. The most common tumors are carcinoma of the lung and breast (Fig 69), leukemia, and lymphoma. With a cytologic examination of the pericardial fluid, the type of malignancy can usually be defined.[29]

Chromosome examination of serous fluid is occasionally helpful in the diagnosis of malignant effusion and adds another dimension to standard cytologic techniques. In one study, an effusion was regarded as malignant when at least three out of thirty metaphase cells were hyperdiploid or contained a marker chromosome.[30]

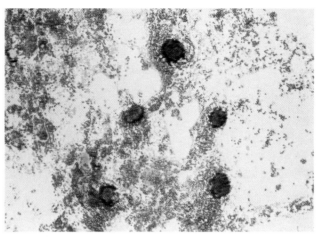

Fig 60.   Characteristic clumping of tumor cells in pleural fluid (low power).

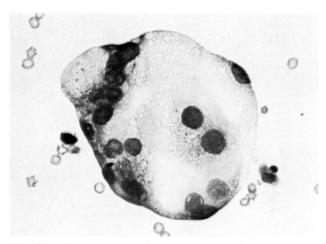

Fig 61.   Bizarre clump of vacuolated cells from the peritoneal fluid of a patient with metastatic ovarian carcinoma.

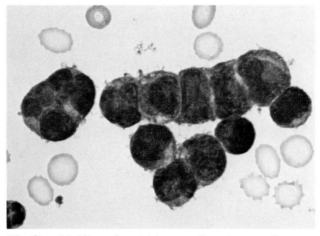

Fig 62.   Molding of nuclei in oat cell carcinoma cells.

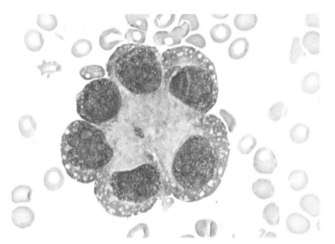

Fig 63. Clump of tumor cells in the pleural fluid of a patient with metastatic breast carcinoma.

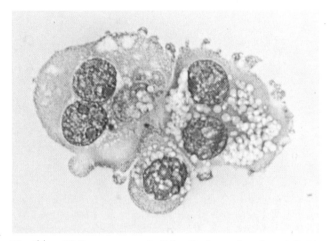

Fig 64. Malignant mesothelial cells from the pleural fluid of a patient with mesothelioma.

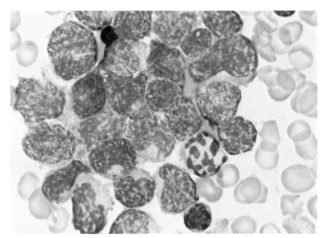

Fig 65. Malignant lymphoma, poorly differentiated lymphocytic type. Note uniform appearance of the malignant lymphocytes.

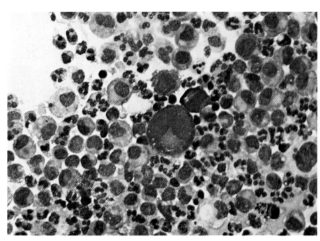

Fig 66. Pleural fluid from a patient with Hodgkin's disease. Note mixed-cell population of neutrophils, histiocytes, lymphocytes, and a Sternberg-Reed cell in the center.

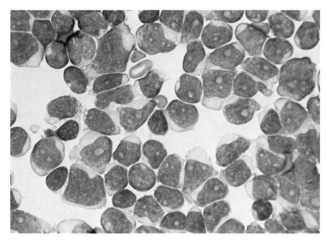

Fig 67. Pleural fluid from a patient with lymphoblastic leukemia. The cells have more cytoplasm than lymphoblasts in the blood, and the nucleoli are more prominent.

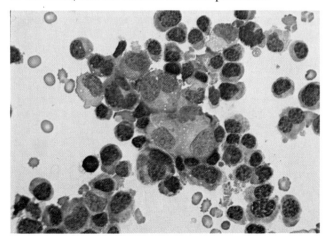

Fig 68. Pleural fluid from a patient with lymphomatoid granulomatosis, revealing lymphocytes at varying stages of transformation, including several large, bizarre lymphoid cells.

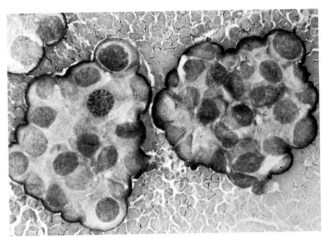

Fig 69. Clumps of tumor cells in pericardial fluid from a patient with metastatic breast carcinoma.

Chemical Analysis

Protein

The value of protein determinations in classifying an effusion according to exudate or transudate was discussed previously. The electrophoretic separation of pleural fluid proteins and quantitation of immunoglobulins do not appear to be of any clinical value.[31]

Glucose

Glucose levels under 60 mg/dl or 40 mg/dl less than the serum glucose are considered decreased.[32] Glucose values less than 30 mg/dl are seen in 70%−80% of the fluids associated with rheumatoid disease,[33] while glucose levels in SLE are usually normal.[34] Pleural fluid glucose levels in malignant effusions, tuberculosis, or empyema may be decreased, although they are more often normal.[32, 35] In effusions associated with congestive heart failure, pulmonary infarction, and those following abdominal surgery, the glucose levels are similar to those in the serum.

Pericardial fluid glucose levels are decreased, in comparison to serum glucose levels, in bacterial endocarditis and malignant effusions.

Acids and Bases

The diagnosis of esophageal rupture usually poses no clinical problem. However, in atypical cases, the diagnosis may be difficult to make. In these situations, the measurement of pleural fluid pH may be helpful. A pleural fluid pH less than 6.0 is suggestive of esophageal rupture.[36]

A pleural fluid pH of 7.3−7.4 is usually "benign" and results in spontaneous resolution, while pH levels below 7.3 are observed with empyema, loculated effusions, and tuberculosis.[37−39] It has been reported that rheumatoid pleural fluids are acidotic and usually have a pH of less than 7.2, while those associated with LE are usually greater than 7.35.[40] In parapneumonic effusions with a pH of less than 7.2, chest tube drainage and antibiotic therapy are recommended.[39] Malignant effusions usually have pH values greater than 7.4. There is generally a good correlation between pleural fluid pH and glucose in parapneumonic effusions.[41]

Blood gas and acid-base measurements appear to be helpful in establishing the origin of bloody pericardial fluid.[42] Simultaneous determinations for pCO_2, pO_2, pH, and bicarbonate on bloody pericardial fluid and arterial blood show a substantial increase in pericardial fluid pCO_2 and a decrease in pericardial fluid pO_2, pH, and bicarbonate when compared to arterial blood.[42]

Enzymes

Pleural fluid *amylase* activity may be increased in a variety of conditions. Levels are considered elevated when they either exceed the normal serum level or are greater than a simultaneously analyzed serum specimen. Since pleural effusions occur in about 10% of the cases with either acute or chronic pancreatitis, amylase determinations may be of assistance in the differential diagnosis.[32] In cases of acute pancreatitis, elevated amylase levels probably are related to lymphatic transport of pancreatic enzymes[28]; while in chronic pancreatitis, the elevated levels are due to internal pancreatic fistulas decompressing into the chest.[43] Since a pleural effusion may be the first sign of pancreatic disease, all unexplained effusions should have amylase activity measured.[32]

Amylase activity may also be increased in pleural effusions secondary to esophageal rupture.[44] It is thought that the elevated amylase levels in these cases are of salivary gland origin.

Malignant effusions have higher *LD* activity than simultaneous serum levels or those seen in benign effusions.[45, 46] Elevated LD levels have also been noted in inflammatory processes, especially when the effusions are highly cellular. In patients with rheumatoid arthritis and SLE, LD activities are moderately elevated but consistently higher in the former.[40]

With the advent of *LD isoenzyme* identification, it was predicted that this technique would be of great assistance in the differential diagnosis of pleural effusions. Subsequent reports, however, have been inconsistent and highly misleading. Some studies have shown that the slower moving bands, LD_4 and LD_5, are increased in malignant effusions, while benign fluids have patterns similar to normal serum with LD_1 and LD_2 predominating.[47, 48] Other studies, however, have shown diametrically opposed patterns for malignant effusions.[49, 50] It appears that this confusion may be related to an inadequate understanding of the pathologic interpretations of the primary lesions, and that the enzyme pattern of the primary tumor cell may be superimposed on secondary cellular elements that alter the measured isoenzyme pattern.[51] Until this information is better understood, LD activity is probably best reserved for separating exudates from transudates.

Alkaline phosphatase activity in pleural effusions associated with pulmonary infarction has been reported to be consistently elevated.[52] In a number of other conditions including malignant effusions, the levels are variable.

Creatine kinase isoenzyme BB (CK-BB) has been recently identified in the serum of patients with various types of cancer. It has been suggested that this isoenzyme represents a tumor-associated marker, particularly for adenocarcinoma of the prostate gland.[53] Effusions secondary to this tumor have demonstrated the presence of the BB isoenzyme.

Lysozyme activity has been noted to be consistently higher in patients with tuberculous pleurisy than in other conditions producing pleural effusions.[54] The measurement of this enzyme may, therefore, be of use in the differential diagnosis of tuberculous effusions.

Other Biochemical Measurements

Zinc, copper, and *iron* have been measured in pleural fluids in both benign and malignant processes.[55] These determinations have, however, no current clinical usefulness. Large amounts of *hyaluronic acid* have been described in pleural and peritoneal fluids from patients with mesotheliomas.[56] Normal levels are considered to be less than 0.8 mg/ml.[28] Glycosaminoglycan electrophoresis of papain digests of mesotheliomas have revealed predominantly hyaluronic acid.[57]

Immunologic Factors

Recent reports indicate that the measurement of *carcinoembryonic antigen (CEA)* in pleural fluid is a valuable adjunct to other methods in detecting malignant effusions.[58, 59] These studies indicate that CEA levels greater than 11−12 ng/ml are almost invariably due to a malignant process. In these studies, when CEA determinations were combined with cytologic findings, the diagnostic accuracy was considerably enhanced.

In addition to the differences in pH and LD activities already mentioned, there are apparent differences in the measurement of *immune complexes* in all fluids from patients with rheumatoid arthritis and SLE. In a recent report,[40] immune complexes were detected in all rheumatoid pleural effusions, using the three assay systems: radioimmunoassay using monoclonal rheumatoid factor, $C1_q$ component of a complement assay, and the Raji cell assay. In most of the rheumatoid fluids, the complexes were detected with all three techniques, and the concentration levels were higher than those simultaneously measured in serum. On the other hand, effusions from patients with SLE were detected primarily by the Raji cell assay, and the pleural fluid concentrations were similar to those measured in serum.[40]

Normal ranges for the *pericardial fluid* complement have recently been determined and are 35−127 mg/dl for C3, 6.3−23.0 mg/dl for C4, and 1.9−9.1 units for the total hemolytic complement (CH50).[60] Pericardial complement levels have been reported to be lower than normal serum values in rheumatoid arthritis and lupus erythematosus.[61, 62]

Microbiologic Examination

Appropriate microbiologic study of pleural fluids for aerobic and anaerobic bacteria is an essential part of the diagnostic workup. All fluids should probably be cultured for aerobic organisms, since these are a more reliable guide to the etiology of the infectious process than sputum cultures. Anaerobic cultures should be carried out if the fluid has a foul odor.

In tuberculous effusions, cultures for acid-fast bacilli are positive in only 25%−50% of the cases. The accuracy can be improved by multiple cultures, by concentrating large volumes of fluid, and by inoculation of guinea pigs. A pleural biopsy is also of recognized value and provides histologic evidence of the disease in 50%– 80% of the cases.[63] Additional information can be obtained when the biopsy specimen is cultured. When these approaches are combined, up to 95% of the cases can be identified.[64]

On rare occasions, fungal, amebic, or echinococcal disease will be seen. In fungal disease, appropriate cultures are usually necessary for accurate diagnosis. In pleuropulmonary involvement with *Entamoeba histolytica,* there is usually an amebic hepatic cyst, and the pleural fluid may show organisms. In hydatid disease, typical hooklets and scolices are readily seen, especially in concentrated specimens.

Counterimmunoelectrophoresis (CIE) for certain bacterial antigens is frequently helpful and may lead to a specific diagnosis within an hour of thoracentesis. The Limulus lysate assay for gram-negative endotoxin is much less reliable for serous effusions than for CSF; improved techniques are needed for this procedure to yield consistently reliable results on pleural fluid.

References

1. Black LF: The pleural space and pleural fluid. Mayo Clin Proc 47:493–506, 1972
2. Sahebjami H, Loudon RG: Pleural effusion: Pathophysiology and clinical features. Sem Roentgenol 12:269–275, 1977
3. Krieg AF: Cerebrospinal fluid and other body fluids, in Henry JB (ed): Clinical Diagnosis and Management by Laboratory Methods, ed 16. Philadelphia: WB Saunders Co, 1979, pp 635–679
4. Light RW, George RB: Incidence and significance of pleural effusion after abdominal surgery. Chest 65:621–625, 1976
5. Light RW, et al: Pleural effusions: The diagnostic separation of transudates and exudates. Ann Intern Med 77:507–513, 1972
6. Teloh HA: The clinical pathology of pleural fluids. Ann Clin Lab Sci 3:98–107, 1973
7. Maher GC, Berger HW: Massive pleural effusion: Malignant and nonmalignant causes in 46 patients. Am Rev Resp Dis 105:458–460, 1972
8. Light RW, Erozan YS, Ball WC: Cells in pleural fluid—Their value in differential diagnosis. Arch Intern Med 854:860, 1973
9. Roy PH, Carr DT, Payne WS: The problem of chylothorax. Mayo Clin Proc 42:457–467, 1967
10. Seriff NS, et al: Chylothorax: Diagnosis by lipoprotein electrophoresis of serum and pleural fluid. Thorax 32:98–100, 1977
11. Dines DE, Pierre RV, Franzen SJ: The value of cells in the pleural fluid in the differential diagnosis. Mayo Clin Proc 50:571–572, 1975
12. Soendergaard K: On the interpretation of atypical cells in pleural and peritoneal effusion. Acta Cytol 21:413–416, 1977
13. Efrati P, Nir E: Morphological and cytochemical investigation of human mesothelial cells from pleural and peritoneal effusions. Isr J Med Sci 12:662–673, 1976
14. Spriggs AI, Boddington MM: The Cytology of Effusions, ed 2. New York: Grune and Stratton Inc, 1968
15. Pettersson T, et al: T and B lymphocytes in pleural effusions. Chest 73:49–51, 1978
16. Bower G: Eosinophilic pleural effusion—A condition with multiple causes. Am Rev Respir Dis 95:746–751, 1967
17. Keshgegian AA: Lupus erythematosus cells in pleural fluid. Am J Clin Pathol 69:570–571, 1978
18. Bynum LJ, Wilson JE: Characteristics of pleural effusions associated with pulmonary embolism. Arch Intern Med 136:159–162, 1976
19. Berger HW, et al: Uremic pleural effusion—A study of 14 patients on chronic dialysis. Ann Intern Med 82:362–364, 1975
20. Galen MA, et al: Hemorrhagic pleural effusion in patients undergoing chronic hemodialysis. Ann Intern Med 82:359–361, 1975
21. Friedman MA, Slater E: Malignant pleural effusions. Cancer Treat Rev 5:49–66, 1978
22. Leff A, Hopewell PC, Costello J: Pleural effusion from malignancy. Ann Intern Med 88:532–537, 1978
23. Billingham ME, et al: The cytodiagnosis of malignant lymphomas and Hodgkin's disease in cerebrospinal, pleural, and ascitic fluids. Cytologica no. 6 (Tokyo) 19:547–556, 1975
24. Weick JK, et al: Pleural effusion in lymphoma. Cancer 31:848–853, 1973
25. Gondos B, et al: Application of electron microscopy in the definitive diagnosis of effusions. Acta Cytol 22:297–304, 1978
26. Domagala W, Woyke S: Transmission and scanning electron microscopic studies of cells in effusions. Acta Cytol 19:214–224, 1974
27. Chandrasekhar AJ, Buehler JH: Diagnostic evaluation of pleural effusion. Geriatrics 29:116–123, 1974
28. Byrd RB: Current concepts in diagnosing the cause of pleural effusion. Geriatrics, 32:44–48, 1977
29. King DT, Nieberg RK: The use of cytology to evaluate pericardial effusions. Ann Clin Lab Sci 9:18–23, 1979

30. Dewald G, et al: Usefulness of chromosome examination in the diagnosis of malignant pleural effusions. N Engl J Med 295:1,494–1,500, 1976

31. Shallenberger DW, Daniel TM: Quantitative determination of several pleural fluid proteins. Am Rev Resp Dis 106:121–122, 1972

32. Light RW, Ball WC Jr: Glucose and amylase in pleural effusions. JAMA 225:257–260, 1973

33. Lillington GA, Carr DT, Mayne JG: Rheumatoid pleurisy with effusion. Arch Intern Med 128:764–768, 1971

34. Carr DT, Lillington GA, Mayne JG: Pleural-fluid glucose in systemic lupus erythematosus. Mayo Clin Proc 45:409–412, 1970

35. Berger HW, Maher G: Decreased glucose concentration in malignant pleural effusions. Am Rev Resp Dis 103:427–429, 1971

36. Dye RA, Laforet EG: Esophageal rupture: Diagnosis by pleural fluid pH. Chest 66:454–456, 1974

37. Funahashi A, Sarkar TK, Kory RC: Measurements of respiratory gases and pH of pleural fluid. Am Rev Resp Dis 108:1,266–1,268, 1973

38. Light RW, et al: Diagnostic significance of pleural fluid pH and pCO_2. Chest 64:591–596, 1973

39. Potts DE, Levin DC, Sahn SA: Pleural fluid pH in parapneumonic effusions. Chest 70:328–331, 1976

40. Halla JT, Schrohenloher RE, Volankis JE: Immune complexes and other laboratory features of pleural effusions. Ann Intern Med 92:748–752, 1980

41. Potts DE, Taryle DA, Sahn SA: The glucose-pH relationship in parapneumonic effusions. Arch Intern Med 138:1,378–1,380, 1978

42. Mann W, Miller JE, Glauser FL: Bloody pericardial fluid. The value of blood gas measurements. JAMA 239:2,151–2,152, 1978

43. Anderson WJ, et al: Chronic pancreatic pleural effusions. Surg Gynecol Obstet 137:827–830, 1973

44. Sherr HP, et al: Origin of pleural fluid amylase in esophageal rupture. Ann Intern Med 76:985–986, 1972

45. Wroblewski F, Wroblewski R: The clinical significance of lactic dehydrogenase activity in serous effusions. Ann Intern Med 48:813–822, 1958

46. Wroblewski F: The significance of alterations in lactic dehydrogenase activity in body fluids in the diagnosis of malignant tumors. Cancer 12:27–39, 1959

47. Richterich R, Zuppinger K, Rossi E: Diagnostic significance of heterogeneous lactic dehydrogenases in malignant effusions. Nature 191:507–508, 1961

48. Richterich R, Burger A: Lactic dehydrogenase isoenzymes in human cancer cells and malignant effusions. Enzymol Biol Clin 3:65–72, 1963

49. Frohlich C, Keller A: LDH-isoenzyme muster in pleuroergussen benigner und maligner atiolgie und ihre diagnostische bedeutung. Klin Wochenschr 45:457–461, 1967

50. Light R, Ball WC Jr: Lactate dehydrogenase isoenzymes in pleural effusions. Am Rev Resp Dis 108:660–664, 1973

51. Griffiths JC: Personal communication

52. Doust JY, Kohout E: Alkaline phosphatase in pleural effusions. Isr J Med Sci 9:1,588–1,590, 1973

53. Silverman LM, et al: Creatine kinase BB: A new tumor-associated marker. Clin Chem 25:1,432–1,435, 1979

54. Klockars M, et al: Pleural fluid lysozyme in human disease. Arch Intern Med 139:73–77, 1979

55. Dines DE, Elvebach LR, McCall JT: Zinc, copper and iron content of pleural fluid in benign and neoplastic disease. Thorax 27:368–370, 1972

56. Hellstrom PE, Friman C, Teppo L: Malignant mesothelioma of 17 years' duration with high pleural fluid concentration of hyaluronate. Scand J Respir Dis 58:97–102, 1977

57. Waxler B, Eisenstein R, Battifora H: Electrophoresis of tissue glycosaminoglycans as an aid in the diagnosis of mesotheliomas. Cancer 44:221–227, 1979

58. Rittgers RS, et al: Carcinoembryonic antigen levels in benign and malignant pleural effusions. Ann Intern Med 88:631–634, 1978

59. Vladutiu AO, Adler RH, Brason FW: Diagnostic value of biochemical analysis of pleural effusions: Carcinoembryonic antigen and Beta$_2$ microglobulin. Am J Clin Pathol 71:210–214, 1979

60. Kinney E, et al: Pericardial-fluid complement. Normal values. Am J Clin Pathol 72:972–973, 1979

61. Richards AJ, et al: Rheumatoid pericarditis: Comparison of immunologic characteristics of pericardial fluid, synovial fluid and serum. J Rheumatol 3:275–282, 1976

62. Goldenberg DL, Left G, Grayzel AI: Pericardial tamponade in systemic lupus erythematosus with absent hemolytic complement activity in pericardial fluid. NY State J Med 75:910–912, 1975

63. Berger HW, Mijia E: Tuberculous pleurisy. Chest 63:88–92, 1973

64. Levine H, et al: Diagnosis of tuberculous pleurisy by culture of pleural biopsy specimen. Arch Intern Med 126:269–271, 1970

3 Peritoneal Fluid

Much of the material discussed in chapter 2 on pleural and pericardial fluid also applies to the examination of peritoneal fluid.

Anatomy and Physiology

The peritoneum is a delicate, smooth, serous membrane that covers the walls and viscera of the abdomen and pelvis. The peritoneum consists of two layers that are contiguous with one another, the space between them forming the *peritoneal cavity*. This cavity is lined by a single layer of mesothelial cells. The two layers of peritoneum are separated by a thin film of fluid that facilitates movement of the two membranes against one another. The peritoneal cavity is not a true cavity, but only becomes so in the presence of disease that leads to an accumulation of fluid within it. The accumulation of fluid within the peritoneal cavity constitutes a peritoneal effusion, and the patient is said to have ascites. The fluid is also called ascitic fluid.

Peritoneal fluid is formed by plasma ultrafiltration. The accumulation of peritoneal fluid may result from increased hydrostatic pressure in the systemic circulation, decreased plasma osmotic pressure, increased permeability of the capillaries in the peritoneum, and decreased lymphatic absorption.

The laboratory criteria for separating transudates from exudates are less clearly defined in peritoneal fluid than pleural fluid. Exudates are usually associated with a protein level of greater than 2.5 gm/dl.[1]

More than 500 ml of peritoneal fluid are usually required before it can be detected by X-ray or physical examination. The major causes of peritoneal effusions are listed in Table 3–1. The indications for aspiration of peritoneal fluid (abdominal paracentesis) are ascites of unknown etiology, suspected intestinal perforation, hemorrhage, or infarct. Aspiration of peritoneal fluid may also be combined with lavage.

Table 3–1. Causes of Peritoneal Effusion*

Transudate
Congestive heart failure
Cirrhosis
Hypoproteinemia

Exudate
Infections (primary or secondary peritonitis)
Neoplasms
Trauma
Pancreatitis

Chylous Effusion
Trauma
Carcinoma
Lymphoma
Tuberculosis
*Adapted from Krieg.[1] Used by permission.

Peritoneal Lavage

The technique of peritoneal lavage consists of inserting a catheter into the peritoneal cavity through a small, midline, infraumbilical incision. If the aspirated fluid reveals free blood, bile-stained fluid, or intestinal content, the test is positive and a laparotomy is indicated. When the test is negative, one liter of normal or balanced saline solution is introduced. Aliquots of the lavage fluid are then examined grossly and sent to the clinical laboratory for hematocrit, RBC and WBC counts, microscopic examination, and chemical and microbiologic evaluations.[2–4]

The indications for peritoneal lavage include combined abdominal and major head injuries, and cases where there is doubt about the extent of intra-abdominal injuries. It is thought to be a reliable indicator of the presence of hemoperitoneum. Contraindications are a gravid uterus, full urinary bladder, and a history of multiple abdominal surgeries.

Gross Examination

Transudates are usually clear and pale yellow. *Exudates* are cloudy or turbid due to large numbers of leukocytes, elevated protein, and occasionally microorganisms. Such fluids may be seen with peritonitis, perforated or infarcted intestine, and pancreatitis. Bile-stained fluid is greenish and may be seen with perforation of the gallbladder or intestine, or duodenal ulcer. Greenish fluid may also be present in cholecystitis and acute pancreatitis. The presence of bile can be confirmed with a "spot" test for bilirubin.[1]

Grossly *hemorrhagic peritoneal fluids* may be seen in trauma (ruptured spleen or liver), intestinal infarction, pancreatitis, and malignancy. Pathologic hemorrhage must be distinguished from a traumatic tap. A visual quantitation of blood in the peritoneal fluid may be useful. The peritoneal lavage method is very sensitive in detecting the presence of blood. As few as eight drops of blood per liter of saline causes pink discoloration.[5] More than 25 ml of blood per liter of lavage fluid gives a bright red, opaque appearance.[2]

True *chylous peritoneal fluid* is rare. When present, it is creamy and has the consistency of milk. Chylous ascites is due to leakage of the thoracic duct from trauma, carcinoma, lymphoma, tuberculosis, and he-patic cirrhosis.[6] Pseudochylous fluid, which may be associated with chronic effusions of any cause, has a milky or greenish appearance due to cellular debris and cholesterol crystals. Methods for differentiating true chylous from pseudochylous fluid are outlined in chapter 2.

Cell Counts

In general, total leukocyte counts are of limited value in the differential diagnosis. A leukocyte count greater than 300 cells/μl is considered abnormal.[7, 8] Counts greater than 500 cells/μl are considered useful in distinguishing peritoneal transudates due to spontaneous bacterial peritonitis from those associated with cirrhosis.[8]

In the presence of abdominal trauma, an RBC count may be particularly valuable. For lavage fluid, more than 100,000 RBCs/μl suggests that there is more than 25 ml of blood per liter in the lavage fluid.[2] In one study, 85% of the patients with lavage fluid RBC counts of 100,000/μl or greater had significant intraperitoneal injury requiring surgical exploration.[4]

Microscopic Examination

A differential count should be performed on a stained smear. The cell types encountered in the peritoneal fluid are the same as those in pleural fluid.[9] For a description of these cells, the reader is referred to chapter 2.

A differential count with greater than 25% *neutrophils* is considered abnormal.[8] A predominance of neutrophils is suggestive of bacterial infection. An absolute neutrophil count is helpful; more than 250 cells/μl is thought to be a fairly sensitive indicator of spontaneous or secondary bacterial peritonitis.[10]

A predominance of *lymphocytes* is seen in transudates due to congestive heart failure, cirrhosis, and nephrotic syndrome. A predominance of lymphocytes may also be seen in chylous effusions, tuberculous peritonitis, and malignancies.

In contrast to pleural fluid, many *mesothelial cells* can occur with tuberculous effusions involving the peritoneal cavity.

Peritoneal fluid *eosinophilia* is less common than pleural fluid eosinophilia. It has, however, been described in association with malignant ascites, ruptured hydatid cyst, congestive heart failure, chronic peritoneal dialysis, and vasculitis.[11]

As with other serous fluids, *lupus erythematosus (LE) cells* have occasionally been reported in peritoneal fluids.[12]

In addition to a differential count, it is important to examine the smear for possible *malignant cells.* When a malignancy is suspected, a specimen should always be examined for cytologic features. With an experienced observer, a cytologic examination is extremely accurate in detecting the presence of malignant cells. The cells that are most difficult to differentiate from malignant ones are mesothelial cells (see chapter 2). Ascitic fluid associated with cirrhosis may contain highly atypical mesothelial cells.[9]

Chemical Analysis

Protein

The measurement of total protein in peritoneal fluid has generally been limited to classifying the fluid as either a transudate or exudate. Classically, fluids containing less than 2.5 gm/dl have been defined as transudates, while those with more than 2.5 gm/dl have been classified as exudates. It is now well known that this is an oversimplification, and that there are many exceptions to this. As a result, the measurement of total protein has limited value in assessing the nature of peritoneal fluid. Multiple measurements, such as those reported for pleural fluids in chapter 2, would probably yield valuable information in this regard.

Tuberculous peritonitis, pancreatic ascites, chronic renal failure, and intra-abdominal neoplasms are usually associated with fluids having protein concentrations of more than 2.5 gm/dl. On the other hand, in spontaneous bacterial peritonitis, the protein concentration reportedly averages 1.8 gm/dl.[13] The fractionation of peritoneal fluid proteins is of little clinical value.

Glucose

The measurement of glucose in peritoneal fluid may be clinically useful in selected cases. The normal levels approximate those found in serum. Unfortunately, few in-depth studies involving a wide variety of disease states have been carried out.

From data currently available, ascitic fluid glucose levels are decreased in 30%–60% of the cases with tuberculous peritonitis and in about 50% of the cases of abdominal carcinomatosis.[14, 15] On the other hand, patients with cirrhosis or congestive heart failure rarely have values below normal. In one study where the blood glucose was simultaneously determined, the blood glucose/ascitic fluid glucose ratio was reportedly 1.0 or greater in 80% of 15 cases with tuberculosis, while all patients with cirrhosis or congestive heart failure had ratios less than 1.0.[14]

Enzymes

An *amylase* determination on peritoneal fluid is often considered part of the complete laboratory examination. Elevations of this enzyme above the normal serum values occur in up to 90% of the cases of acute or traumatic pancreatitis, or pancreatic pseudocyst. However, increased ascitic fluid amylase activity is not limited to these conditions but has been reported in 77% of 26 patients with gastroduodenal perforation,[16] in acute mesenteric venous occlusion,[17] and in small bowel strangulation with or without perforation.[18]

More recently, ascitic fluid *lipase* has been measured and considered complementary to, and perhaps more reliable than, amylase in the diagnosis of pancreatic ascites.[19] These authors reported significantly increased lipase activity over normal serum levels. In addition, they suggested that lipase activity may fluctuate less than amylase activity and may remain within a narrow range.

Alkaline phosphatase (ALP) activity is very high in the intestinal tract. Several studies have shown that the measurement of ALP in peritoneal fluid may be helpful in evaluating certain patients with abdominal disorders.[20–22] Patients with bowel strangulation, intestinal perforation, or traumatic hemoperitoneum may have greatly elevated peritoneal fluid ALP levels in comparison to serum ALP levels. In these conditions, other enzymes, notably *lactate dehydrogenase (LD)* and *aldolase,* are also elevated but are less specific than ALP.

In isolated traumatic liver injuries both serum and peritoneal fluid may show marked elevations of *aspartate aminotransferase (AST, GOT),*[22] *alanine aminotransferase (ALT, GPT),* and LD.

The LD activity is usually elevated in malignant abdominal effusions when compared with simultaneously determined serum levels. Benign effusions usually have values comparable to or lower than those in the serum. However, peritoneal fluid LD activity has been studied in much less detail than in pleural effusions. It is probable, as with pleural fluids, that attempts to interpret these results, including the isoenzymes, will be confusing and yield little helpful information at this time.

Gamma-glutamyl transferase (GGT) levels in ascitic fluid have been reported to be markedly increased in patients with primary hepatoma.[23] In comparison, peritoneal fluids from a variety of other hepatic disorders including metastatic carcinoma have shown greatly decreased levels. Only in cases of active cirrhosis with cellular regeneration have the GGT levels been mildly elevated, as compared to other hepatic disorders.[23]

Other Biochemical Measurements

Ammonia levels in peritoneal fluid have been shown to be consistently increased over simultaneous plasma levels in cases of ruptured appendix, perforated peptic ulcer, bowel strangulation with or without perforation, and ruptured urinary bladder with extravasation of urine.[24, 25] Ammonia values are normal in pancreatitis.

Blood urea nitrogen (BUN) and *creatinine* measurements are sometimes used to differentiate between peritoneal fluid and urine. Elevated levels of BUN and creatinine in the fluid with normal serum values indicate aspiration from the urinary bladder. Elevated BUN and creatinine in the fluid with a high serum BUN but normal serum creatinine suggest rupture of the bladder.

Lactic acid has been reported to be increased in the peritoneal fluid of animals with ischemic bowel disease.[26] In addition, experimentally induced intestinal ischemia in dogs has resulted in a significant rise in peritoneal fluid lactic acid levels.[21]

Early diagnosis and treatment of intestinal infarction is a difficult clinical problem, the mortality approaching 90% when necrosis is extensive. It has been suggested, however, that early diagnosis is possible using the appropriate clinical techniques, since these patients frequently have elevated serum and peritoneal fluid phosphorus levels, metabolic acidosis, and leukocytosis.[27]

Several studies have shown that the boardlike abdomen characteristic of peptic ulcer perforation is not due to acid-peritonitis. The *pH* of the peritoneal fluid following perforation is actually alkaline in practically all cases and is due to rapid neutralization of the liberated gastric acid.[28, 29] As a result, pH measurements of ascitic fluid have little diagnostic value.

Carcinoembryonic Antigen

The diagnostic value of carcinoembryonic antigen (CEA) measurements in ascitic fluid has been recently evaluated.[30] In "benign" ascites, the levels were consistently less than 10 ng/ml. Fluids with CEA levels greater than 10 ng/ml were considered to represent malignant effusions. Using these criteria, CEA measurements accurately detected 14 of 29 malignant effusions, while a cytologic examination detected only 12.[30] The combined use of cytologic and CEA measurements resulted in an accurate diagnosis in 20 of 29 cases.[30]

Microbiologic Examination

The diagnosis of *tuberculous peritonitis* is often difficult and frequently overlooked, since the classic features of prolonged fever, weight loss, exudative ascites, and a positive tuberculin skin test may not always be present. Of assistance in these cases is the fact that in tuberculous peritonitis, ascitic fluid protein levels usually exceed 2.5 gm/dl, and glucose values are less than 60 mg/dl; or the simultaneous blood glucose/ascitic fluid glucose ratio is 1.0 or greater.[14] When either or both of these findings are present, appropriate cultures for tubercle bacilli should be requested. A peritoneal biopsy may be of diagnostic significance.

Spontaneous bacterial peritonitis (SBP) is a relatively common disease, and in patients with cirrhosis, the mortality is high (80%–95%).[8] The ascitic fluid is cloudy, and the WBC count (predominantly polymorphonuclear) is usually above 1,000/μl. A Gram's stain of the centrifuged specimen is helpful, and organisms can frequently be seen. In about two thirds of these cases, gram-negative bacilli are present, while pneumococci account for most of the remaining cases. In contrast to tuberculous peritonitis, the protein content in SBP is usually less than 2.5 gm/dl.[13]

Counterimmunoelectrophoresis (CIE) for bacterial antigens may be extremely useful, just as it is for other body fluids. On the other hand, Limulus lysate assays are less reliable for peritoneal fluid than for CSF. Further studies and improved techniques are needed before the latter procedure becomes routine with peritoneal or pleural fluids.

References

1. Krieg AF: Cerebrospinal fluid and other body fluids, in Henry JB (ed), Clinical Diagnosis and Management by Laboratory Methods, ed 16. Philadelphia: WB Saunders Co, 1979, pp 635–679
2. Olsen WR, Redman HC, Hildreth DH: Quantitative peritoneal lavage in blunt abdominal trauma. Arch Surg 104:536–543, 1972
3. Jergens ME: Peritoneal lavage. Am J Surgery 133:365–369, 1977
4. Engrav LH, et al: Diagnostic peritoneal lavage in blunt abdominal trauma. J Trauma 15:854–859, 1975
5. Parvin S, et al: Effectiveness of peritoneal lavage in blunt abdominal trauma. Ann Surg 181:255–261, 1975
6. Lesser GT, Bruno MS, Enselberg K: Chylous ascites. Arch Intern Med 125:1,073–1,077, 1970
7. Kline MM, McCallum RW, Guth PH: The clinical value of ascitic fluid culture and leukocyte count studies in alcoholic liver disease. Gastroenterology 70:408–412, 1976
8. Conn HO: Spontaneous bacterial peritonitis. Multiple revisitations. Gastroenterology 70:455–457, 1976
9. Spriggs AI, Boddington MM: The Cytology of Effusions, ed 2. New York: Grune and Stratton Inc, 1968
10. Jones SR: The absolute granulocyte count in ascitic fluid—An aid to the diagnosis of spontaneous bacterial peritonitis. West J Med 126:344–346, 1977
11. Adams HW, Mainz DL: Eosinophilic ascites. Am J Dig Dis 22:40–43, 1977
12. Metzger AL, Coyne M, Lee S: In vivo LE cell formation in peritonitis due to SLE. J Rheumatol 1:130, 1974
13. Conn HO, Fessel JM: Spontaneous bacterial peritonitis in cirrhosis: Variations on a theme. Medicine (Baltimore) 50:161–197, 1971
14. Polak M, Torres DaCosta AC: Diagnostic value of the estimation of glucose in ascitic fluid. Digestion 8:347–352, 1973
15. Brown JD, An ND: Tuberculous peritonitis. Am J Gastroenterol 66:277–282, 1976
16. Amerson JR, Howard JM, Vowles KDJ: The amylase concentration in serum and peritoneal fluid following perforation of gastroduodenal ulcers. Ann Surg 147:245–250, 1958
17. Gray EB Jr, Amador E: Acute mesenteric venous thrombosis simulating acute pancreatitis. The value of peritoneal fluid analysis. JAMA 167:1,734–1,736, 1958
18. Mansberger AR Jr: The diagnostic value of abdominal paracentesis with special reference to peritoneal fluid ammonia levels. Am J Gastroenterol 42:150–161, 1964
19. Sileo AV, Chawla SK, LoPresti PA: Pancreatic ascites: Diagnostic importance of ascitic lipase. Dig Dis Sci 20:1,110–1,114, 1975
20. Lee YN: Alkaline phosphatase in intestinal perforation. JAMA 208:361, 1969
21. Rush BF Jr, et al: Intestinal ischemia and some organic substances in serum and abdominal fluid. Arch Surg 105:151–157, 1972
22. Delaney HM, Moss CM, Carnevale N: The use of enzyme analysis of peritoneal blood in the clinical assessment of abdominal organ injury. Surg Gynecol Obstet 142:161–167, 1976
23. Peters TJ, et al: Gamma-glutamyltransferase levels in ascitic fluid and liver tissue from patients with primary hepatoma. Br Med J 1:1,516, 1977
24. Mansberger AR Jr: The value of peritoneal fluid ammonia levels in the differential diagnosis of the acute abdomen. Ann Surg 155:998–1,010, 1962
25. Mansberger AR Jr: The diagnostic value of abdominal paracentesis with special reference to peritoneal fluid levels. Am J Gastroenterol 42:150–161, 1964
26. Moore JN, et al: Lactic acid concentration in peritoneal fluid of normal and diseased horses. Res Vet Sci 23:117–118, 1977
27. Sower BA, Jamieson WG, Durand D: The significance of elevated peritoneal fluid phosphate level in intestinal infarction. Surg Gynecol Obstet 146:43–45, 1978
28. Moretz WH, Erickson WG: Neutralization of hydrochloric acid in the peritoneal cavity. Arch Surg 75:834–837, 1957
29. Howard JM, Singh LM: Peritoneal fluid pH after perforation of peptic ulcers. Arch Surg 87:483–484, 1963
30. Loewenstein MS, et al: Carcinoembryonic antigen assay of ascites and detection of malignancy. Ann Intern Med 88:635–638, 1978

4 Synovial Fluid

Analysis of synovial fluid plays a major role in the diagnosis of joint disease. When infective arthritis and crystal-induced synovitis are suspected, examination of synovial fluid may produce a definitive diagnosis. These two conditions, therefore, are the most important indications for arthrocentesis and synovial fluid analysis; but in all other diseases, a diagnosis may not be possible from synovial fluid examination alone. However, the categorization of common joint diseases can usually be accomplished on the basis of synovial fluid analysis. Thus, the results may indicate whether an effusion is inflammatory or noninflammatory, and whether hemarthrosis is present. Normal adult reference values for the components of synovial fluid are presented in Table 4–1.

Table 4–1. Normal Adult Reference Values for Synovial Fluid*

Components	Conventional Units	SI Units
Glucose (blood-synovial fluid difference)	0–10 mg/dl	<0.55 mmole/liter
Leukocyte count	0–200/μl	0–0.20 × 10^9/liter
Neutrophils	<25%	<0.25
Protein	1–3 gm/dl	10–30 gm/liter

*Adapted from Krieg.[1] Used by permission.

Anatomy and Physiology

Diarthrodial joints are lined at their margins by synovium, a tissue consisting of synovial cells lining the joint space. These cells have the capacity for protein synthesis and phagocytosis. The underlying connective and adipose tissues are supplied by a rich vascular network.

Synovial fluid is basically an ultrafiltrate of the plasma combined with a mucopolysaccharide (hyaluronate) that is synthesized by the cells of the synovial membrane.[2] The functions of the synovial fluid are to lubricate the joint space and transport nutrients to the articular cartilage. The protein and immunoglobulin levels of the synovial fluid are approximately one fourth that of plasma, while the glucose and uric acid concentrations are the same as the blood levels.

Mechanical, chemical, or bacteriologic damage may alter the permeability of the membranes and capillaries to produce varying degrees of inflammatory response. Various disorders produce changes in the chemical constituents of the joint fluid and in the type of cell population present.

Through clinical and laboratory examination of the joint fluid, joint disorders can be divided into five categories (Table 4–2). This classification is useful as long as it is realized that there may be considerable overlap in synovial fluid findings among the different groups. The five major disease categories are: Group I—noninflammatory, Group II—inflammatory, Group III—infectious, Group IV—crystal-induced, and Group V—hemorrhagic.[3]

Impaired function of the synovial fluid with age or disease may play a role in the development of degenerative joint disease (osteoarthritis). Inflammatory joint fluids contain lytic enzymes that produce depolymerization of hyaluronic acid, which markedly impairs the lubricating ability of the fluid.

Sample Collection and Detection

There are no absolute contraindications to joint aspiration. The incidence of septic complications is exceedingly low when the procedure is performed by an experienced practitioner using aseptic precautions. Relative contraindications are the presence of local sepsis such as cellulitis, bacteremia, and a congenital or acquired bleeding tendency. The technique of aspiration has been well described in recent publications.[2, 4]

For routine examination, the syringe used for removing the fluid should be moistened with an anticoagulant (approximately 25 units heparin/1 ml synovial fluid).[5] Oxalate and powdered ethylenediaminotetraacetic acid (EDTA) should not be used because they can produce artifacts in the microscopic examination for crystals. When adequate fluid is available, it should ideally be divided into three samples. Approximately 3 ml are collected in a sterile tube for microbiologic examination, 5 ml are collected in an anticoagulated tube (heparin or liquid EDTA) for microscopic examination, and

the remainder is placed in a plain tube and allowed to clot (normal fluid does not clot). The specimen is then centrifuged to remove all cells. Cells in the synovial fluid may alter the chemical composition of the fluid; therefore, centrifugation should not be delayed. This is particularly important when complement levels are desired.[2] The supernatant can be used for assay of rheumatoid factor, antinuclear antibody, complement levels, immunologic substances, and chemicals. It is important that for complement determinations, the test should be performed within 2-3 hours since the complement is heat-labile. If immediate examination cannot be accomplished, the fluid should be frozen and stored at -70 C until examined.

When the synovial fluid is unusually viscid, the high viscosity may cause difficulty in the performance of several tests. The fluid may be digested with hyaluronidase for a period of several hours prior to the analysis.[6]

If the arthrocentesis reveals a dry tap, there may still be a few drops of fluid within the needle that can be used for a culture or microscopic examination. One should, therefore, not discard the needle but leave it on the syringe and transport it to the laboratory inserted into a sterile cork.

When only a small amount of fluid is obtained during arthrocentesis, it may be difficult to decide whether it represents synovial fluid, fluid from subcutaneous tissue, or the local anesthetic. Mucin formation and metachromatic staining are two methods used for detecting as little as 0.5 ml of synovial fluid.[7] The *mucin clot test* consists of precipitating any mucin present with 2% acetic acid, followed by an examination for the presence of turbidity or a mucin clot.

The *metachromatic staining* procedure consists of spotting filter paper with synovial fluid and then staining

Table 4-2. Classification of Arthritides*

Group I Noninflammatory	Group II Inflammatory	Group III Infectious	Group IV Crystal-induced	Group V Hemorrhagic
Osteoarthrosis	Rheumatoid arthritis	Bacterial	Gout	Traumatic arthritis
Traumatic arthritis	Lupus erythematosus	Mycobacterial	Pseudogout	Hemophilic arthropathy
Osteochondritis dissecans	Reiter's syndrome	Fungal		Anticoagulation
Osteochondromatosis	Rheumatic fever			Pigmented villonodular
Neuropathic osteoarthropathy	Ankylosing spondylitis			synovitis
Pigmented villonodular	Regional enteritis			Neuropathic osteoarthropathy
synovitis	Ulcerative colitis			Synovial hemangioma
	Psoriasis			

*Adapted from Rippey.[3] Used by permission.

with a few drops of 0.2% aqueous toluidine blue. Metachromasia of the synovial fluid spots is seen after a few seconds. The metachromatic staining procedure is probably the most sensitive method, but it is not suitable for analysis of fluid that has been in contact with heparin, since heparin is strongly metachromatic with toluidine blue.

Gross Examination

The analysis of synovial fluid starts with recording the volume and the gross appearance of the removed fluid. Effusions of all arthritides produce variable volumes of synovial fluid. There is little correlation among the volume, etiology, and severity of the joint disease.

Normal fluid is light yellow, clear, and does not clot. Hemorrhagic fluid is homogeneously bloody. In a traumatic aspirate, streaks of blood are seen. Centrifugation of the fluid may be necessary to differentiate between a traumatic tap and hemarthrosis. Xanthochromia of the supernatant usually indicates that blood has been present in the synovial fluid for some time. Xanthochromia may, however, be difficult to interpret because of the normal light yellow color of synovial fluid. A dark red or brown supernatant in the presence of gross blood suggests hemarthrosis rather than a traumatic tap. Turbidity usually indicates leukocytosis and increases with the degree of inflammation. Other factors that may produce a turbid fluid include cartilage debris or the presence of crystals. Fluid from a joint with crystal-induced synovitis (gout and pseudogout) may be purulent and milky, and occasionally greenish. Cloudy and fatty fluid usually indicates the presence of cholesterol crystals, often seen in chronic arthritides. The presence of clear, pale yellow, viscous fluid usually indicates a noninflammatory disease from Group I. Fluid from Group II inflammatory diseases is frequently turbid, yellow, and clots while standing. Fluid from a patient with Group III infectious diseases is grossly purulent.

As previously noted, normal synovial fluid does not clot. However, in the presence of an inflammatory condition, fibrinogen and other coagulation factors are present, and clot formation does occur.

Cell Counts

The reported upper limit of normal for the leukocyte count in synovial fluid varies considerably from less than 200/μl to less than 750/μl.[1] However, most authors consider 200/μl as the upper limit of normal.[4] The leukocyte count may be performed in a standard hemocytometer or in a Fuchs-Rosenthal chamber.[2] Electronic counting equipment may also be used. Unless the leukocyte count is very high ($> 50,000$/μl), the total count can be performed with undiluted fluid.[1] Physiologic saline should be used as a diluent instead of one containing acetic acid, since the latter will precipitate hyaluronic acid and produce cell clumping. It is important that the fluid be properly agitated before being added to the counting chamber. This can be done by using a bench vibratory mixer.[1] When the fluid is highly viscous, it may need to stand in the hemocytometer for more than 30 minutes before the cells settle and can be counted.[1] The addition of hyaluronidase in phosphate buffer reduces the viscosity of the synovial fluid, makes it easier to pipet, and allows a more even cell distribution in the counting chamber.

The total leukocyte count can be performed using either a phase-contrast microscope or a standard light microscope. When the latter is used, 0.1% methylene blue is helpful in identifying the leukocytes.[1, 2]

When the fluid is heavily contaminated with blood, the RBCs should be lysed using a diluent such as the absolute basophil diluent or hypotonic saline (see Appendix). The RBCs should, however, also be counted, unless it is clear that they originate from a traumatic tap.

The total leukocyte count is of some use in categorizing the fluid into one of the five disease groups described before (see Table 4–2). Therefore, in septic arthritis the leukocyte count is almost always greater than 50,000/μl.[8] It should be noted, however, that there may be considerable overlap in all ranges, and that the leukocyte count is not diagnostic by itself. For example, in the early phase of bacterial infection, the leukocyte count may be normal. In addition, occasional cases of gout or rheumatoid arthritis (RA) may have leukocyte counts in the range usually associated with septic arthritis.[8]

Differential Count

The differential count can be made by phase-contrast microscopy at the time of the leukocyte count, although a more accurate one is obtained by using a Wright's stained smear of concentrated (centrifuged) synovial fluid. It is important that the films be made thin, since staining of the mucopolysaccharide and mucoproteins in the synovial fluid may obscure the cell morphology.[2]

A high percentage of neutrophils (>80%) is highly suggestive of septic arthritis regardless of the magnitude of the total leukocyte count. When the percentage of neutrophils is markedly elevated, a Gram's stain and a search for intracellular bacteria are recommended.

In RA of less than six weeks' duration, lymphocytes are the initial, predominant cell type.[9] Later, there is a predominance of neutrophils.[8] There have been occasional reports of acute gout and acute pseudogout without synovial fluid leukocytosis, suggesting an alternative inflammatory mechanism.[10]

In one study, 70% of the patients with culture-proven infectious arthritis had leukocyte counts above 50,000/µl, while 12.5% of the patients with gout, 10% of those with pseudogout, and 4% of those with rheumatoid arthritis also had leukocyte counts in this range.[8] In one fourth of the fluids containing uric acid crystals and one third of the fluids with calcium pyrophosphate crystals, the leukocyte counts were below 2,555/µl.[8] This emphasizes the need for a careful search for crystals in fluids with high as well as low leukocyte counts. It is also important to note that septic arthritis can coexist with other types of arthritis such as gout, pseudogout, systemic lupus erythematosus (SLE), and RA.[1]

Cell Morphology

Normal synovial fluid contains approximately 65% mononuclear phagocytes, a variable number of lymphocytes, and less than 25% neutrophils.[5] No cartilaginous or inclusion-bearing cells are normally seen, and polarized light microscopic examination reveals no crystals. The number of RBCs varies and may result from a traumatic tap.

The types of cells that may be seen in a microscopic examination of abnormal synovial fluid include neutrophils, lymphocytes, plasma cells, monocytes, macrophages, synovial lining cells, and lupus erythematosus (LE) cells. Neutrophils and lymphocytes generally show a morphologic structure identical to that of the corresponding cells of the blood (Figs 70 and 71). The *neutrophils* may contain vacuoles, fat droplets, bacteria, or crystals. Commonly, the nucleus shows pyknosis and karyorrhexis. The *mononuclear phagocytes,* which include monocytes, macrophages, and histiocytes (Fig 72),

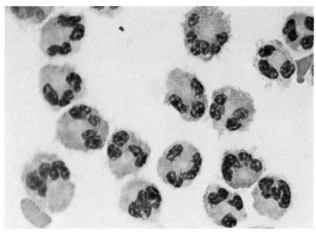

Fig 70. Numerous neutrophils in synovial fluid, as seen in bacterial arthritis.

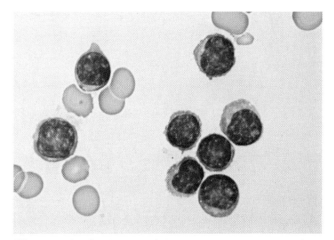

Fig 71. Predominance of lymphocytes in synovial fluid from a patient with Felty's syndrome.

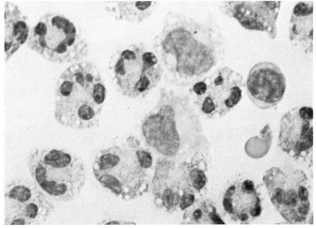

Fig 72. Two histiocytes, a lymphocyte, and several neutrophils in synovial fluid.

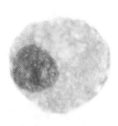

Fig 73. A single synovial lining cell.

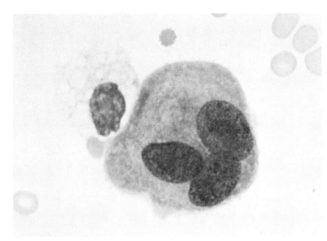

Fig 74. A multinucleated synovial lining cell resembling a mesothelial cell.

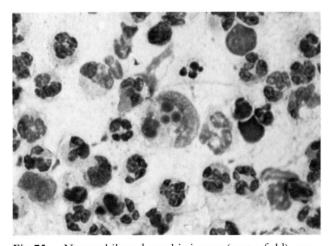

Fig 75. Neutrophils and two histiocytes (center field), containing bluish, intracytoplasmic inclusions that are probably ingested neutrophils, from a patient with Reiter's syndrome.

may be similar to blood monocytes but often show a variable morphology and may be difficult to differentiate from the *synovial lining cells* (Fig 73). These latter cells also resemble mesothelial cells (Fig 74). The presence of synovial lining cells does not appear to have any specific diagnostic significance.[2]

So-called *Reiter cells* are vacuolated macrophages containing either neutrophilic or basophilic globular material, or both (Fig 75). Such cells, however, are not specific for Reiter's disease.[11] *Ragocytes* or *RA cells* are neutrophils containing small, dark, cytoplasmic granules that are best identified with phase-contrast microscopy.[2, 4, 5] Immunofluorescent techniques have shown that these inclusions consist of immune complexes such as IgG, IgM, complement, and rheumatoid factor. The RA cells are not specific for RA and may also be seen in gout and septic arthritis.[12] Occasionally, *LE cells* may be seen in synovial fluid from patients with lupus erythematosus, and some cases have been reported in which LE cells are initially present in the synovial fluid and not in the peripheral blood (Fig 76). Some LE cells may also be seen in synovial fluid from patients with RA.[1]

Giant, multinucleated *cartilage cells* are typically seen in osteoarthritis, but isolated cartilage cells may appear in a number of arthridites.[5, 13] In pigmented villonodular synovitis, the presence of *papillary aggregates* of *synovial cells* is a characteristic finding, and hemosiderin inclusions are often found within synovial cells.[13] Many multinucleated foreign-bodied giant cells may also be seen.[5] In *ochronosis*, which refers to the accumulation of melanin-like pigment in connective tissues of persons with alkaptonuria, one may see synovial fluid speckled with dark particles resembling ground pepper. Microscopic examination of this fluid has revealed fragments of pigmented cartilage.[14]

Crystals

Examination of synovial fluid for crystals using polarized light should be done routinely. Specimens with or without anticoagulants may be used. However, as mentioned before, powdered EDTA or oxalate should not be used as an anticoagulant, since both may be associated with crystal formation. Ideally, a wet preparation of the fluid should be examined immediately to demonstrate intracellular crystals. Birefringent crystals are also readily demonstrated in thin, dried smears when many crystals are present, as may be seen in acute gout.

It is important to have a polarizing microscope of excellent quality to properly examine the specimen. This is particularly true with calcium pyrophosphate crystals, which are weakly birefringent and may be missed unless the polarizing equipment is adequate. Polarized light, using a polarizer and an analyzer, allows one to make a diagnosis of crystal-induced arthritis. However, the definitive identification of the type of crystal, ie, urate and/or calcium pyrophosphate dihydrate, requires the addition of a first order *red compensator* (Fig 77). The red compensator is a retardation plate that alters the passage of light into slow and fast components. When inserted between the polarizer and analyzer, it retards the polarized light so that the field background becomes red instead of black.[1, 2, 15, 16]

The types of crystals that may be seen in synovial fluid include uric acid, calcium pyrophosphate dihydrate, cholesterol, steroid, and apatite.

The presence of *uric acid* crystals is usually a diagnostic indication of gout.[17] These crystals may be intracellular or extracellular, or both, are needle-like with pointed ends, and measure $1-20$ μ in length (Fig 78). The presence of intracellular crystals should be noted in the laboratory report, since this indicates the acute stage of gout. If only extracellular crystals are found, it is unlikely that these are responsible for the acute symptoms. Uric acid crystals are seen in approximately 90% of the patients during an acute attack of gout. Between acute attacks, they may be seen in approximately 75% of the patients.[1] In a small number of patients, even during an acute attack, uric acid crystals may not be found.[18, 19] The reasons for this include aspiration from the wrong site, loculation within the joint, crystal dissolution, examiner inexperience, and insufficient search for crystals.[19] Therefore, repeated examinations for uric acid crystals may be required occasionally for a definitive diagnosis.

Under polarized light, uric acid crystals are strongly birefringent, ie, they appear bright against a dark, fully polarized background (Fig 79). Using a red compensator, they are yellow when their longitudinal axis is parallel to the slow component of the compensator (Fig 80). The crystals are then considered negatively birefringent.[1, 2, 15, 16]

Calcium pyrophosphate dihydrate crystals, which are associated with pseudogout, are rod-like, plate-like, or rhomboid. These crystals appear pale against the dark background of polarized light, ie, they are weakly birefringent and may be overlooked by the inexperienced observer (Fig 81). They may also appear as needles and

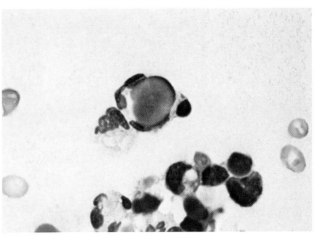

Fig 76. An LE cell in the synovial fluid from a patient with lupus erythematosus.

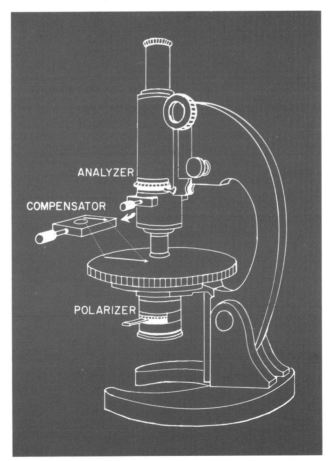

Fig 77. Polarizing equipment used for crystal detection in synovial fluid.

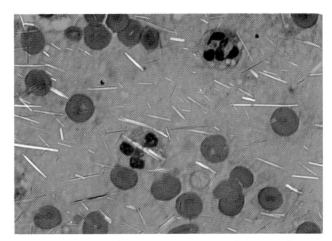

Fig 78.   Intra- and extracellular uric acid crystals from a patient with acute gout (polarized light).

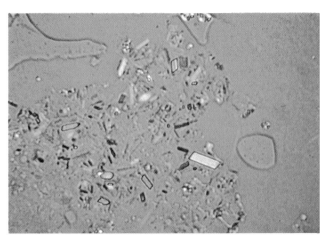

Fig 81.   Calcium pyrophosphate crystals in synovial fluid from a patient with pseudogout (polarized light).

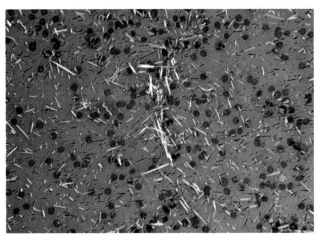

Fig 79.   Multiple uric acid crystals in synovial fluid from a patient with gout (polarized light).

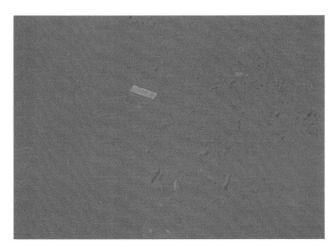

Fig 82.   Calcium pyrophosphate crystals from a patient with pseudogout. Their characteristic colors also depend on the crystals' orientation to the compensator's axis (polarized light with red compensator).

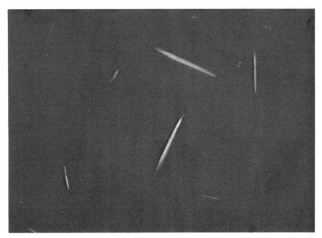

Fig 80.   Uric acid crystals from a patient with gout. Note characteristic colors that depend on the orientation of the crystals to the compensator's axis (polarized light with compensator).

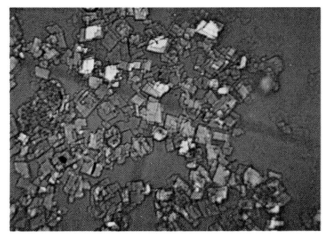

Fig 83.   Cholesterol crystals from a patient with chronic rheumatoid arthritis (polarized light). From Kitridou.[20] Used by permission.

be mistaken for uric acid crystals. Using a red compensator, calcium pyrophosphate crystals have a blue color when their longitudinal axis is parallel to the slow component of the compensator (Fig 82). They are then considered to be positively birefringent.

Leukocyte counts of 65,000–100,000/µl with >90% neutrophils have been found in synovial fluids from patients with gout and pseudogout. This may cause confusion with infectious arthritis and points out the importance of routinely examining all synovial fluids for crystals.[8]

Cholesterol crystals are usually shaped like rectangular, notched plates (Fig 83).[20] They are considered to be nonspecific and are seen in chronically inflamed joints such as those associated with RA.

Corticosteroid preparations used for intra-articular injections are suspensions of microcrystals that may be similar in size and shape to uric acid and calcium pyrophosphate crystals.[1, 21] The microcrystals may be present for as long as a month after injection. It is, therefore, essential to know whether the patient has received a recent injection of corticosteroids.

Arthritis—particularly osteoarthritis—is occasionally associated with *apatite* crystals. They appear as shiny inclusions in wet preparations or as dark purple, cytoplasmic neutrophil inclusions with Wright's stain.[22] Electron microscopy may be required for a definitive identification.

Artifacts that may be mistaken for crystals include collagen fibrils, pieces of cartilage, scratches and dirt on the glass slide, and phagocytosed metal or plastic materials in joints containing prostheses.

Chemical Analysis

In the past, the chemical analysis of synovial fluid, if performed at all, consisted of measuring glucose and occasionally total protein. Other rough indicators of disease, still frequently performed, are the mucin and fibrin clot evaluations. The mucin clot test essentially determines the state of the hyaluronic acid-protein complex and, hence, is related to viscosity. Both mucin clot formation and hyaluronic acid concentration are generally decreased in inflammatory conditions. Fibrin clot formation is simply the observation of spontaneous clotting. Normally, synovial fluid does not clot, since fibrinogen and other clotting factors are absent. Inflammatory and bloody fluids both produce spontaneous clotting.

Considerably more diagnostic information on the chemical and immunologic composition of synovial fluid is now available. Although much of this information has little clinical significance, there are several helpful tests in selected patients. Most of the chemical and immunologic tests carried out on serum can be applied equally well to synovial fluid. If viscosity presents a technical problem, this can usually be overcome by appropriate dilution of the specimen or by prior sonication; or pretreatment with the enzyme, hyaluronidase, is effective (0.9 ml synovial fluid incubated for four hours at 37 C with 0.1 ml bovine testicular hyaluronidase).

Hyaluronic Acid

Hyaluronic acid, a copolymer of glucuronic acid and N-acetyl-glucosamine, is secreted by the synovial lining cells and imparts to the fluid its stickiness and high viscosity. The normal mean concentration is about 0.41%.[12] Its concentration is decreased in old age as well as in postmortem fluid. The molecular weight and concentration of hyaluronic acid are reduced in inflammatory joint diseases. There is, however, no clinical significance to its specific routine measurement.

Protein

The normal synovial fluid protein concentration is approximately one third that of serum with an average of about 2.0 gm/dl.[1] Levels above 3.0 gm/dl suggest an inflammatory or hemorrhagic exudate. The quantitative methods used for measuring total serum protein are satisfactory for synovial fluid. The protein concentration of synovial fluid depends upon synovial membrane permeability, synovial fluid resorption by lymphatics, the molecular weight of the various protein molecules, and local synthesis.[1] Increased levels are routinely seen in RA, gout, septic arthritis, SLE, the inflammatory arthropathies accompanying Crohn's disease, Reiter's disease, ankylosing spondylitis, psoriasis, and ulcerative colitis. Most of these proteins are derived from plasma due to increased vascular permeability. There is also local immunoglobulin synthesis.

Clinically, the finding of an elevated total protein merely confirms the presence of an inflammatory process, which is information usually obtained from other observations. Protein electrophoresis adds little useful clinical information.

Glucose

The measurement of synovial fluid glucose may be of clinical value but is not specific. Similar to CSF, synovial fluid levels are interpreted along with serum values. Ideally, to establish an equilibrium, the synovial and serum levels are obtained 6–8 hours postprandially; but this is usually impossible from a practical viewpoint. The synovial fluid glucose level is normally equal to or slightly below (within 10 mg/dl) the serum level. In general, noninflammatory joint disorders (degenerative joint disease, neuropathic osteoarthropathy, pigmented villonodular synovitis, trauma, and so forth) have levels less than 20 mg/dl below the simultaneous serum levels. Inflammatory joint diseases (rheumatoid arthritis, rheumatic fever, SLE, and Reiter's disease, among others) have levels greater than 25 mg/dl below the serum levels. In cases of septic arthritis, the synovial fluid glucose level is often more than 40 mg/dl below the serum concentration (Table 4–3).[3] There is, however, considerable overlap in the levels between noninflammatory joint disorders and septic arthritis.

Uric Acid

Although the diagnosis of gout can often be made by synovial fluid crystal identification, misinterpretations can occur. This is particularly true when the examiner is relatively inexperienced, or the proper polarizing equipment is not available.

The quantitation of synovial fluid uric acid levels will not only verify the presence of uric acid crystals but may also be diagnostically significant even when no crystals are found. It has been suggested that the synovial fluid uric acid concentration is a better, single diagnostic factor than the serum level.[23] Normally, synovial fluid and serum uric acid concentrations are similar. A synovial fluid uric acid concentration significantly above the normal serum level is probably diagnostic of gout.[6] In untreated gout, both synovial fluid and serum levels of uric acid are usually elevated. It should be mentioned, however, that some investigators believe that uric acid measurement in synovial fluid has little or no diagnostic value.[1,4]

Enzymes

Many enzymes have been studied in synovial fluid including lactate dehydrogenase (LD), aspartate aminotransferase (AST, GOT), acid and alkaline phosphatase, muramidase (lysozyme), β-acetyl-glucosaminidase, and 5′-nucleotidase, among others.

Synovial fluid—but not serum—LD levels are increased in patients with RA, infectious arthritis, and gout.[24] The LD activity is normal in synovial fluid from patients with osteoarthritis. Isoenzyme patterns of synovial fluid in patients with RA, infectious arthritis, and gout show a predominance of LD_5.[24] This isoenzyme is probably derived from neutrophils that are usually abundant in all of these disorders, especially during the acute phase. On the other hand, AST (GOT) was normal in all cases in the same study.[24]

Table 4–3. Synovial Fluid Findings*

	Normal	Group I Noninflammatory	Group II Inflammatory	Group III Infectious	Group IV Crystal-Induced	Group V Hemorrhagic
Appearance	yellow, clear	yellow, clear, slightly cloudy	yellow, cloudy	yellow, green, turbid-bloody	yellow, turbid-milky	red-brown, xanthochromic
White cell count (per μl)	0–200	0–5,000	2,000–100,000	50,000–200,000	500–200,000	50–10,000
PMNs (%)	<25	<30	>50	>90	<90	<50
Crystals	no	no	no	no	yes	no
RBCs	no	no	no	yes	no	yes
Glucose (blood-synovial fluid difference in mg/dl)	0–10	0–10	0–40	20–100	0–80	0–20
Culture	negative	negative	negative	often positive	negative	negative

*Adapted from Krieg[1] and Rippey.[3]

Considerable interest has been expressed regarding the action of acid hydrolases as destructive agents in rheumatoid joint disorders. Studies of both acid phosphatase and β-acetyl-glucosaminidase have been carried out.[25-27] They have shown elevations of both enzymes, with the highest values being seen in RA. Nevertheless, increased activity is not specific for this entity. It is postulated that the acid phosphatase originates from polymorphonuclear leukocytes (PMNs). Alkaline phosphatase, although present in synovial fluid, is not elevated in any of the inflammatory arthropathies. Enzyme activity appears to be related primarily to the degree of synovial inflammation. Their routine measurement apparently adds no additional useful clinical information that is not obtained from more routine examinations.

Other Biochemical Measurements

Many other substances have been measured in synovial fluid in normal and diseased joints. For example, the concentration of *iron* has been found to be consistently elevated in both the synovial fluid and synovial membranes of patients with RA.[28] The levels are usually greater than the corresponding serum concentrations. Increased iron deposition in synovium also occurs in hemochromatosis and pigmented villonodular synovitis. *Zinc* is present in the synovial fluid of patients with RA in greater concentration than is found in serum.[29] Although these studies are interesting, they have little clinical usefulness.

Synovial effusions containing *cholesterol* crystals have been described in several types of chronic arthritides and are particularly common in RA.[30, 31] The fluids have a turbid, white or yellow, thick consistency. Quantitative synovial fluid cholesterol levels are usually considerably greater than those in the serum and may be diagnostically significant. Triglyceride levels are invariably in the normal serum range.

Immunologic Evaluation

Normal synovial fluid contains only about 10% of the *immunoglobulin* levels of normal serum. Mild increases occur in crystal synovitis and degenerative joint disease. In RA and related disorders, the immunoglobulin levels approach those in serum. In classic RA with nodules, Cracchiolo and Barnett,[32] using radial immunodiffusion (RID), reported that the synovial fluid/serum ratios for IgG, IgA, and IgM averaged 0.7. The ratios of those cases without nodules were 0.5, as were the "probable" RA cases. Patients with osteoarthritis had mean ratios of 0.3. In seven cases of Reiter's syndrome, the synovial fluid/serum ratio for IgM approached 1.4, the IgA ratio averaged 1.0, and the IgG ratio averaged 0.85. This was the only disease in which the ratios consistently exceeded 1.0.

Rheumatoid factors (RF) are most often detected by the agglutination of sensitized sheep RBCs, bentonite, or latex particles coated with γ-globulin. These tests are semiquantitative and do not indicate the distribution of the anti-γ-globulins among the different classes. Only IgM rheumatoid factor is measured by these tests. Methods for the detection of IgG and IgA rheumatoid factors are generally considered to be research tools. The latex fixation test appears to be the most sensitive, but can lead to a few false-positive results. While the sensitized sheep RBC agglutination test appears less sensitive, it may be more specific.[32] In about 80% of the patients with RA, rheumatoid factors are present in the serum. In approximately 60% of the patients, RF can be detected in synovial fluid.[32] Occasional seronegative patients will test positive for RF in synovial fluid.[32-34] Since a wide variety of other chronic inflammatory processes are characterized by persistent antigenic stimuli, false-positive results are common.[33-35] In general, assays for RF in synovial fluid have not been helpful for diagnosis or prognosis.[36]

Antinuclear antibodies (ANA) are immunoglobulins with specific antibody activity against antigens in cell nuclei. They occur in all three classes of immunoglobulins and can be detected by the same methods used for serum. Nearly all patients with active SLE will have detectable ANA in their sera, while 10%–65% of the patients with RA will be ANA-positive depending on the sensitivity of the test used.[37] Approximately 70% of the patients with SLE will have ANA in the synovial fluid, while about 20% of the RA patients will be positive for ANA.[4, 32] There is, however, little disease specificity associated with synovial ANA.[36]

Complement components are a group of nonspecific serum factors that interact in a specific sequence during immunologic reactions. The synovial fluid determination of total hemolytic complement (CH50), which measures the ability of the fluid to lyse 50% of a standard suspension of sheep erythrocytes coated with rabbit antibody, may be helpful in selected patients.

Synovial fluid complement levels correlate well with

total protein concentration.[38] As a result, interpretation depends not only on the total complement level but also on the total protein. Bunch et al[38] have reported the following normal values:

Total Protein (mg/ml)	Complement (units/ml)
20	8–38
30	11–42
40	15–46
50	19–50

From this information, appropriate interpolations can be made for other protein-complement values. It should be noted that in this report, the normal serum range was reported as 40–90 CH50 units/ml. In another study, the reference level of synovial total complement suggested that normal values are more than 30% of the simultaneous serum value.[35] It is possible that C_4 is a more sensitive index than total complement.[39]

Total synovial fluid complement is normal in traumatic or degenerative joint disease. However, decreased levels are usually seen in SLE, RA, and bacterial synovitis. Levels may be elevated in Reiter's disease.[11] Serum complement levels are usually decreased in SLE, particularly in patients with renal disease, and are normal or increased in RA (Table 4–4). Panush et al[40] have reported a linear relationship between elevated serum or synovial fluid IgG and IgM anti-γ-globulins and lowered serum or synovial fluid complement. Hence, an elevation of serum and synovial fluid for complement and RF may be helpful in difficult or unusual cases.

It should be noted that complement is heat-labile and unless the test can be performed within two to three hours, the specimen should be rapidly frozen.

Table 4–4.   Complement Levels in Joint Disease

Disease	Serum	Synovial Fluid
Rheumatoid arthritis	Normal or increased	Normal or decreased
Systemic lupus erythematosus	Normal or decreased	Decreased
Reiter's disease	Increased	Increased
Gout	Increased	Increased

Microbiologic Evaluation

The routine examination of synovial fluid should include a Gram's stain and culture for microorganisms. Occasionally, other studies are needed. Because of this, careful thought about the etiologic possibilities should precede the aspiration of a joint effusion. Consultation with an appropriate laboratorian may save a great deal of time and lead to a correct diagnosis that otherwise might be missed. Even in cases of arthritis of presumedly known noninfectious origin, it must be kept in mind that a secondary bacterial infection is possible. In addition, in early or mild bacterial infections, the gross examination of the fluid may suggest a nonseptic etiology. Failure to culture the specimen may result in a missed or delayed diagnosis, a prolonged clinical course, and possible permanent injury to the joint.

Although viruses, tuberculosis, and fungi may all be possible causative agents, bacteria are clearly the most common infectious organisms. They usually reach the synovial membrane from the blood stream. Hence, the epidemiology of infectious arthritis is essentially that of bacteremia.

The age of the patient is critical and gives important clues to the specific organism one might expect to recover.[41] In young children, systemic infections such as pneumonia or meningitis are commonly present with infectious arthritis. The most common organisms are *Staphylococcus aureus*, *Streptococcus pyogenes*, *Streptococcus pneumoniae*, and *Hemophilus influenzae*. The last organism is seen almost exclusively in children under 2 years of age. In children 2–15 years of age, *S aureus*, *S pyogenes*, and *S pneumoniae* account for about 85% of the cases. Regarding ages 16–50, *Neisseria gonorrhoeae* accounts for 75% of the cases, and *S aureus* for 15%. In patients over 50 years of age, gonococci are rarely seen, and *S aureus* accounts for up to 75% of the cases; the remaining 25% is composed of a variety of different bacteria.

The enteric organisms are only occasionally isolated as causative agents. Although they are most frequently seen in patients over 50 years of age, they account for no more than 10%. Microorganisms other than those already mentioned collectively account for less than 5% of the cases in any age group.

Since *N gonorrhoeae* is so important as a causative agent, it is imperative that the proper media be inoculated immediately after aspiration of the fluid. Due to the fastidious nature of this organism, the appropriate prewarmed culture media should be immediately available. If tuberculosis, fungi, or anaerobic bacteria are suspected, special handling and culture media are also needed. Prior consultation with the laboratory is again very helpful. In the case of tuberculosis, a closed synovial biopsy for histologic examination, using a Parker-Pearson needle or similar technique, may provide the diagnosis.

In addition to the usual studies, synovial fluid can be examined by counterimmunoelectrophoresis (CIE) for specific bacterial antigens, as well as for endotoxin by the Limulus lysate assay (see chapter 1). These techniques give rapid, reliable, and specific information in selected cases.

References

1. Krieg AF: Cerebrospinal fluid and other body fluids, in Henry JB (ed): Clinical Diagnosis and Management by Laboratory Methods, ed 16. Philadelphia: WB Saunders Co, 1979, pp 635–657

2. Currey HLF, Roberts BV: Examination of synovial fluid. Clinics in Rheumatic Diseases 2:149–176, 1976

3. Rippey JH: Synovial fluid analysis. Lab Med 10:140–145, 1979

4. Cohen AS, Brandt KD, Krey PR: Synovial fluid, in Cohen AS (ed): Laboratory Diagnostic Procedures in the Rheumatic Diseases. Boston: Little Brown and Co, 1975

5. Naib ZM: Cytology of synovial fluids. Acta Cytol 17:299–309, 1973

6. Teloh HA: Clinical pathology of synovial fluid. Ann Clin Lab Sci 5:282–287, 1975

7. Goldenberg DL, Brandt KD, Cohen AS: Rapid, simple detection of trace amounts of synovial fluid. Arth Rheum 16:487–490, 1973

8. Krey PR, Bailen DA: Synovial fluid leukocytosis, a study of extremes. Am J Med 67:436–442, 1979

9. Gatter RA, Richmond JD: Predominance of synovial fluid lymphocytes in early rheumatoid arthritis. J Rheumatol 2:340–345, 1975

10. Matthay M, et al: Acute pseudogout in the absence of synovial fluid leukocytes. J Rheumatol 4:303–306, 1977

11. Pekin TJ, Malinin TI, Zvaifler NJ: Unusual synovial fluid findings in Reiter's syndrome. Ann Intern Med 66:677–684, 1967

12. Stafford CT et al: Studies on the concentration and intrinsic viscosity of hyaluronic acid in synovial fluids of patients with rheumatic diseases. Ann Rheum Dis 23:152–157, 1964

13. Broderick PA, et al: Exfoliative cytology interpretation of synovial fluid in joint disease. J Bone Joint Surg [Am] 58:396–399, 1976

14. Hunter T, Gordon DA, Ogryslo MA: The ground pepper sign of synovial fluid: A new diagnostic feature of ochronosis. J Rheumatol 1:45–53, 1974

15. Phelps P, Steele AD, McCarty DJ: Compensated polarized light microscopy. JAMA 203:166–179, 1968

16. Yehia SR, Duncan H: Synovial fluid analysis. Clin Orthop 107:11–24, 1975

17. McCarty DJ, Hollander JL: Identification of urate crystals in gouty synovial fluid. Ann Intern Med 54:452–460, 1961

18. Romanoff NR, et al: Gout without crystals on initial synovial fluid analysis. Postgrad Med J 54:95–97, 1978

19. Schumacher HR, et al: Acute gouty arthritis without urate crystals identified on initial examination of synovial fluid, report on nine patients. Arthritis Rheum 18:603–612, 1975

20. Kitridou RC: Synovianalysis. Am Fam Physician 5:101–107, 1972

21. Kahn CB, Hollander JL, Schumacher HR: Corticosteroid crystals in synovial fluid. JAMA 211:807–809, 1970

22. Schumacher HR, et al: Arthritis associated with apatite crystals. Ann Intern Med 87:411–413, 1977

23. Reeves B: Significance of joint fluid uric acid levels in gout. Ann Rheum Dis 24:569–571, 1965

24. Cohen AS: Lactic dehydrogenase (LDH) and transaminase (GOT) activity of synovial fluid and serum in rheumatic disease states, with a note on synovial fluid LDH isozymes. Arthritis Rheum 7:490–501, 1964

25. Lehman MA, Kream J, Brogna D: Acid and alkaline phosphatase activity in the serum and synovial fluid of patients with arthritis. J Bone Joint Surg [Am] 46:1,732–1,738, 1964

26. Caygill JC, Pitkeathly DA: A study of β-acetylglucosaminase and acid phosphatase in pathological joint fluids. Ann Rheum Dis 25:137–144, 1966

27. Veys EM, et al: N-acetyl-β-D-glucosaminidase activity in synovial fluid. Rheumatol Rehabil 14:50–56, 1975

28. Senator GB, Muirden KD: Concentration of iron in synovial membrane, synovial fluid, and serum in rheumatoid arthritis and other joint diseases. Ann Rheum Dis 27:49–53, 1968

29. Castor CW, Prince RK, Hazelton MJ: Hyaluronic acid in human synovial effusions; a sensitive indicator of altered connective tissue cell function during inflammation. Arthritis Rheum 9:783–794, 1966

30. Meyers OL, Watermeyer GS: Cholesterol-rich synovial effusions. S Afr Med J 50:973–975, 1976

31. Ettlinger RE, Hunder GG: Synovial effusions containing cholesterol crystals. Mayo Clin Proc 54:366–374, 1979

32. Cracchiolo A, Barnett EV: The role of immunological tests in routine synovial fluid analysis. J Bone Joint Surg [Am] 54:828–840, 1972

33. Rodnap GP, Eisenbeis CH, Creighton AS: The occurrence of rheumatoid factor in synovial fluid. Am J Med 35:182–188, 1963

34. Huskisson EC, Hart FD, Lacey BW: Synovial fluid Waaler-Rose and latex tests. Ann Rheum Dis 30:67–72, 1971

35. Seward CW, Osterland CK: The pattern of anti-immunoglobulin activities in serum, pleural and synovial fluids. J Lab Clin Med 81:230–240, 1973

36. McCarty DJ Jr: Synovial fluid, in Hollander JL, McCarty DJ Jr (eds): Arthritis and Allied Conditions. A Textbook of Rheumatology. Philadelphia: Lea & Febiger, 1979, pp 51–69

37. Cracchiolo A: Joint fluid analysis. Am Fam Physician 4:87–94, 1971

38. Bunch TW, et al: Synovial fluid complement determination as a diagnostic aid in inflammatory joint disease. Mayo Clin Proc 49:715–720, 1974

39. Ruddy S, Austen KF: The complement system in rheumatoid synovitis. I. An analysis of complement component activities in rheumatoid synovial fluids. Arthritis Rheum 13:713–723, 1970

40. Panush RS, Bianco NE, Schur PH: Serum and synovial fluid IgG, IgA and IgM antigammaglobulins in rheumatoid arthritis. Arthritis Rheum 14:737–747, 1971

41. Parker RH: Septic arthritis, in Hoeprich PD (ed): Infectious Diseases, ed 2. New York: Harper & Row, 1977, pp 1,125–1,132

Appendix: Laboratory Methods

The methods for obtaining extravascular body fluids are considerably more complicated than those for collecting a peripheral blood specimen. The process is potentially dangerous and usually uncomfortable for the patient. These fluids should, therefore, be handled and examined with great care.

Fluid Collection

Ideally, the specimens should be collected in three separate allotments with each tube labeled in the order that it is obtained. If a microbiologic examination is indicated, the specimen must be submitted in a sterile tube. The second or third tube is recommended for the cell count and microscopic examination, since contamination with peripheral blood is less likely in these tubes.

Since most serous fluids will clot, the specimen should be anticoagulated immediately. However, an anticoagulant should not be added to the CSF.

All fluids should be sent to the laboratory as soon as possible and examined promptly. The CSF should always be examined immediately and handled as a "stat" specimen. Lysis of cells in the CSF takes place soon after removal from the body. Even though all body fluids should be examined as soon as possible, satisfactory smears can be made up to 24 hours after collection of pleural, peritoneal, and synovial fluids. Fluids containing large numbers of RBCs show more rapid cell deterioration than clear fluids.

Body fluids submitted for special cytologic examination should be diluted 1:1 with 50% alcohol fixative. Smears made from body fluids should be "cyto-fixed" (spray fixative).

The routine analysis of body fluids consists of (1) gross examination, (2) total cell count, (3) differential count and search for abnormal cells and crystals, (4) microbiologic examination, (5) chemical analysis, (6) immunologic examination, and (7) cytologic examination. Several of the methods used for the various laboratory examinations have been mentioned in the main text or referred to in the references. In this appendix, we will describe in detail the more commonly used laboratory methods for analysis of body fluids.

Manual Cell Count

Diluents

The following diluents may be used for cell counts:

1. Saline. (Both WBCs and RBCs are preserved.)
2. Gower's solution for RBCs. (Add 12.5 gm of sodium sulfate to 33.3 ml of glacial acetic acid diluted with water to 200 ml.)*
3. Türk's solution for WBCs. (Add 3 ml of acetic acid to 1 ml of 1% gentian violet diluted with water to 100 ml.)*
4. Buffered diluent
   a. Weigh and place the following in a 250-ml Erlenmeyer flask: 0.1 gm of dextrose, 0.02 gm of toluidine blue O, and 0.025 gm of hyaluronidase (Type 1-S†).
   b. Prepare buffer solutions
      1. Add 2.279 gm of potassium phosphate monobasic (0.067 M), qs to 250 ml with distilled water.
      2. Add 9.511 gm of sodium phosphate dibasic (0.067 M), qs to 1,000 ml with distilled water.
   c. Add the following and swirl to mix well: 6.5 ml of potassium phosphate monobasic (0.067 M), 43.5 ml of sodium phosphate dibasic (0.067 M), and 6.5 ml of absolute methanol.
   d. Store counting diluent in refrigerator in a tightly stoppered bottle. Filter before use. It is stable for about two months.
5. Absolute basophil diluent
   a. This diluent is particularly useful for grossly bloody specimens. It lyses the RBCs and stains the WBCs.
   b. Dissolve 1.05 gm of toluidine blue O in 100 ml of 0.85% saline.
   c. Make a saturated solution of saponin in 50% methanol, and allow excess saponin to settle until clear; do not centrifuge or filter.
   d. Mix together 40 ml of toluidine blue O solution, 11 ml of absolute methanol, and 1 ml of saponin solution. Store in refrigerator, and filter before use with slow-speed paper.
   e. Other methods for lysing RBCs include dilution with 0.3% saline, 0.1 N hydrochloride, or 1% saponin in saline.

---

*These solutions contain acetic acid that will clump mucin and fluids with a high protein content. They should not be used in synovial fluids.

†Sigma Chemical Company, Saint Louis, MO 63178.

Comments

Synovial fluids that are often highly viscous or mucoid may be difficult to work with. Addition of hyaluronidase in phosphate buffer will reduce the viscosity, making the fluid easier to pipet and resulting in a more even cell distribution. Add 1 drop of 0.05% hyaluronidase in phosphate buffer to each milliliter of synovial fluid, mix, and wait four minutes; then dilute with buffered diluent, described previously.

Clotting of the fluid invalidates the results of a cell count. If the fluid clots, the clinician should be notified of this immediately. Do not, however, discard the specimen. If the clinician still insists on having the cell count done, it should be noted on the report that the specimen was clotted. A laboratory procedure to follow in analyzing body fluids is illustrated in Figure 84.

Cell Count in a Hemocytometer

1. Fluid should be flooded on the chamber while still undiluted after having been thoroughly mixed, using an improved Neubauer hemocytometer or Fuchs-Rosenthal counting chamber and covered with a thick coverslip. Both sides of the hemocytometer should be filled with fluid and counted to assure accuracy.
2. If the fluid is not too thick (ie, there is no overlapping of cells), count the undiluted specimen. Count the RBCs and WBCs on both sides of the chamber, and take an average of the two counts.
3. If the cells are too numerous to count, the fluid must be diluted according to the number of cells present using an RBC or WBC pipet, eg, 1:10, 1:100. Let the dilutions stand in the pipet for 5–10 minutes before putting fluid in chamber.
   a. When counting RBCs, dilute with Gower's solution or saline. These diluents do not remove the WBCs.
   b. When counting WBCs, use Türk's solution or buffered diluent.
4. With grossly bloody fluids, RBCs may be lysed with absolute basophil diluent prior to the white cell count. For red cell counts, a dilution of 1:100 or 1:200 is made with cell counting diluent.
5. The number of cells present determine the area to be counted (Fig 85).
   a. If there are numerous cells, count those in the smaller squares in the center of the chamber

(RBC area). By counting these smaller areas, a smaller number of cells are counted. Count five RBC squares.

b. If the cells are less numerous, the larger four WBC areas of the chamber may be counted.

c. When only a few cells are present, the entire chamber should be counted.

6. Cells as they appear in the hemocytometer:

RBCs: distinct outline with halo and clear centers. If crenated, they have many fine-pointed projections.

WBCs: granular appearance.

Tissue cells: usually appear as large granular cells with irregular outlines. Broken cells or tissues cells are not included in the total count.

Note: Cell counts should always be verified by Wright's stained smears.

7. Calculation of results should be based on the following formula: Total cells/μl =

$$\frac{\text{no. of cells} \times \text{dilution}}{\text{no. of squares counted} \times \text{volume of each square}}$$

This formula represents only one of the many methods used for calculating results.

8. Examples, using:

RBC square volume = 0.004 μl
WBC square volume = 0.1 μl
Entire chamber volume = 0.9 μl

a. Thirty RBCs were found in five squares of the red cell-counting area when the fluid was diluted 1:10.

$$\frac{30 \times 10}{5 \times 0.004} = 15,000 \text{ RBC}/\mu l$$

b. One hundred twenty WBCs were found in the four white cell-counting areas on an undiluted fluid.

$$\frac{120 \times 1}{4 \times 0.1} = 300 \text{ WBC}/\mu l$$

c. Twenty-five WBCs were counted on the entire chamber on an undiluted fluid.

$$\frac{25 \times 1}{1 \times 0.9} = 28 \text{ WBC}/\mu l$$

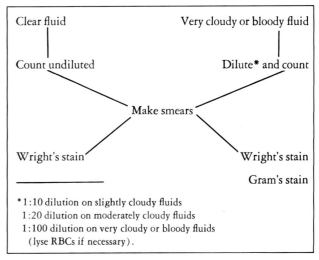

Fig 84. Laboratory procedure to follow in analyzing clear fluids as differentiated from very cloudy or bloody fluids.

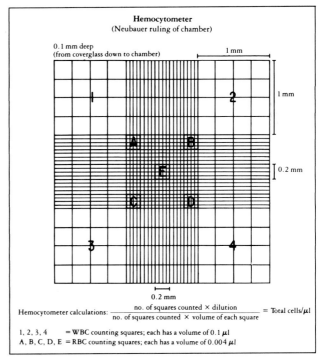

Fig 85. Neubauer hemocytometer for counting RBCs and WBCs.

Electronic Cell Count

Electronic cell counters are not used for the CSF since the background counts cause poor precision in the normal range. Also, several investigators recommend that electronic counting equipment should not be used for any serous fluid since cellular debris may cause false elevation of the cell count. Nevertheless, many laboratories use Coulter* counters routinely for pleural and peritoneal fluids.

We have found a good correlation between leukocyte counts, using the hemocytometer and the Coulter counter model S, when the leukocyte count is above 1,000 cells/μl. The Coulter counter model F^n or ZBI should be used for RBC counts and is also probably more accurate for leukocyte counts.

Direct aspiration through the sample valve on a Coulter model S is recommended unless the fluid is viscous or contains fibrin clots. If the fluid is viscous or contains clots, or only a small amount of fluid is received, make a 1:224 dilution (44.7 μl fluid plus 10 ml Isoton*), and bypass the sampling valve by use of a microsampler.

With the Coulter model F^n and ZBI, use a 1:500 dilution for WBCs and RBCs.

It must be remembered that the electronic counters count all cells including tissue cells. Therefore, the count may have to be adjusted, depending on the cell types seen in smears.

Differential Count

A differential count should be performed on stained smears made from concentrated leukocytes and not in the hemocytometer. Numerous methods have been described for concentrating the cells in body fluids. These include centrifugation with smears made from the resuspended sediment, sedimentation methods,[1-5] cytocentrifugation,[6-8] and filtration.[5]

Ordinary centrifugation with staining of the sediment, the routine of the past, has the advantage of requiring no special equipment. There is, however, a variable recovery of cells with this method, and considerable cellular damage occurs during centrifugation with resultant difficulty in preparing good quality smears.

The filter techniques using Millipore,* Nucleopore,† or Gelman‡ filters give excellent recovery of cells. However, it is more time consuming than some of the other methods, and considerably more skill is required to prepare a satisfactory specimen. The cytocentrifuge method has many advantages and is now commonly used. The cell yield is satisfactory, though not as good as with filter techniques. However, due to the speed and simplicity, the cytocentriguge method is superior to other concentration methods. In addition, 12 samples can be processed simultaneously. It is particularly useful for a large laboratory. However, the centrifugation produces some distortion of the cell morphology.

Several sedimentation methods have been described that provide excellent morphology, but the cell yield is usually not as good, and it is more time consuming than the cytocentrifuge method.

Cytocentrifuge§ Method

Depending upon the appearance and type of fluid, varied amounts may be used: clear fluid, 5–10 drops; cloudy fluid, 1–3 drops. When the fluid is bloody, a 1:5 dilution with saline is used. When it is grossly bloody, use a push smear. Figure 86 depicts the cytocentrifuge instrument.

1. Place the cytocentrifuge cups into the centrifuge opposite each other. Smears should be made in duplicate.
2. Label the slides with patient's name, hospital number, date, and type of fluid.
3. Place special filter paper against a glass slide in back of the cup, making certain the hole in the cup lines up with the hole in the carrier (Fig 87).
4. Put the drops of fluid into the cup with a Pasteur pipet (Fig 88).
5. Add 2 drops of 22% albumin to reduce the cell distortion and to increase the yield.
6. Lock the lid into position, and spin at 1,000 rpm for 5–10 minutes.
7. Carefully remove the slides and filter papers together. Mark a circle around the concentrate on the back of the slide with a red crayon (Fig 89).
8. Air-dry slides before staining.

---

*Coulter Electronics, Inc, Hialeah, FL 33010.

*Millipore Corporation, Bedford, MA 01730.
†Nucleopore, Fairfax, CA 94930.
‡Gelman Instrument Company, Ann Arbor, MI 48106.
§Shandon Southern Instruments Inc, Sewickley, PA 15143.

9. Stain the slides with Wright's stain or other stains when indicated, and coverslip (Fig 90).
10. Do a differential count. If possible, count 100 cells; if not, count as many cells that are found on the concentrate. Mesothelial cells and macrophages may or may not be included in the differential count.
11. Cytocentrifuge cups should be cleaned in soapy water, rinsed well in tap water, distilled water, and finally, in isopropyl alcohol. They are air-dried.

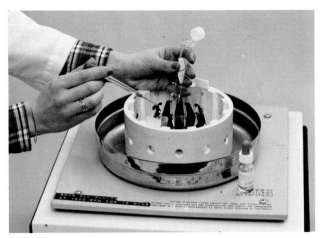

Fig 88. Drops of fluid are added to the cytocentrifuge cup.

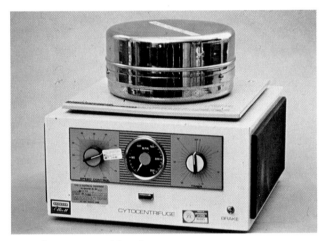

Fig 86. Cytocentrifuge instrument.

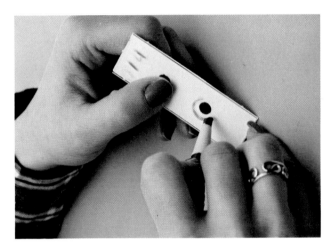

Fig 89. The back of the glass slide is marked with a red crayon to indicate the area of cell concentrate.

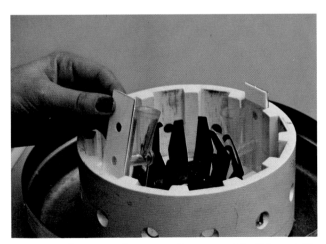

Fig 87. Placement of cytocentrifuge cup with slide and filter paper into the centrifuge.

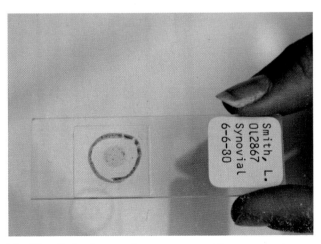

Fig 90. Stained smear from a cytocentrifuge preparation.

Comments

Variable cellular distortion is frequently seen with the cytocentrifuge method. The cells near the center are smaller with denser nuclear chromatin than those at the periphery. Nuclear and cytoplasmic distortion may be seen, especially the latter with the formation of irregular cytoplasmic processes (Fig 91). Other artifacts occasionally encountered are the peripheral localization of nuclear lobes in polymorphonuclear leukocytes (Fig 92), an acidophilic or amphophilic paranuclear zone in mononuclear cells, peripheral cytoplasmic vacuolation, localization of cytoplasmic granules, and holes in the nuclei (Fig 93). These cellular distortions are, however, not usually troublesome to an experienced observer.

To delay fluid absorption and increase cellular yield, a small amount of immersion oil may be spread around the hole of the filter paper (1 cm in diameter) prior to centrifugation.

The speed and time of centrifugation can be varied, depending on the type of fluid, to insure maximum cell yield and optimum cell preservation.

Sedimentation Method

Equipment needed for the sedimentation method[1] is featured in Figure 94.

1. Punch a round hole approximately 1 cm in diameter in the center of a stack of 9-cm Whatman* no. 2 filter papers.
2. Wrap one filter paper around one long edge of a microscopic slide in such a manner that the hole will be in the center of the slide.
3. Transfer 0.2–1.0 ml of fresh fluid into a disposable plastic cup,† 1.8 ml in capacity. The amount of fluid used depends upon cell concentration.
4. Place the wrapped slide on top of the cup with the hole in the paper in the center of the mouth of the cup.
5. Hold the cup and slide together with one hand, and use the other hand to slide the no. 18 ball-and-socket joint pinch clamp‡ sideways with one blade on the clamp above the microscopic slide, and the other beneath the ledge around the lip of the cup.

*W & R, Balston, England.
†Matheson Scientific Co, Elk Grove Village, IL 60007.
‡Arthur H. Thomas Co, Philadelphia, PA 10105.

6. After the cup and the slide are secured, turn the entire set-up over so that the cup is inverted (Fig 95). Allow to settle for 20–30 minutes. The fluid is absorbed by the filter paper, and the cells settle on the exposed surface of the slide. The more fluid there is, the longer it takes to absorb.
7. When the cup is dry, remove the slide and allow to dry in the air for a few minutes (Fig 96).
8. Stain the slide.

Comments

Many types of sedimentation methods have been described, particularly for use in CSF cytology.[1–5]

Examination of Synovial Fluid for Crystals

Uric acid crystals are diagnostic of gout, while calcium pyrophosphate crystals are seen in pseudogout. Cholesterol crystals are nonspecific and correlate well with the chronicity of the arthritis. Steroid crystals are occasionally seen in joints previously injected with steroids.[9]

Synovial fluid should be viewed in a relatively fresh state. A small drop is placed on a glass slide. A coverslip is placed over the top and sealed with Vaseline or nail polish to delay drying. The glass slide and coverslip should be cleaned with alcohol and dried with clean gauze prior to the examination. Crystals may also be seen in stained smears but with greater difficulty.

The specimens should be examined with a good polarizing microscope. Such a microscope contains two prisms or filters: (1) the polarizer that is situated below the condenser and (2) the analyzer that is located above the objective. A first-order red compensator is placed between the polarizer and the analyzer. The first-order red compensator separates light into components of slow and fast vibration.

The specimen is first examined with polarized light, without the red compensator, using the high dry objective. The light source is increased to maximum, and the polarizer or analyzer is rotated into position, making the field as dark as possible. Uric acid crystals appear as strongly birefringent rods or needles varying 1–20 μ in length. The urate crystals from a tophus may be very large. They may be intracellular or extracellular.

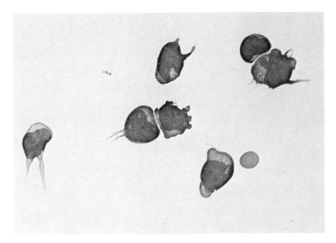

Fig 91. Cytoplasmic processes from several blast cells in the CSF. These processes represent artifacts produced by centrifugation.

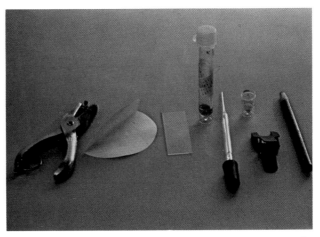

Fig 94. Equipment used for concentrating cells in the sedimentation method.

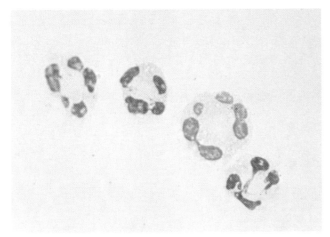

Fig 92. An example of cellular distortion seen with the cytocentrifuge method—peripheral localization of nuclear segments in CSF neutrophils.

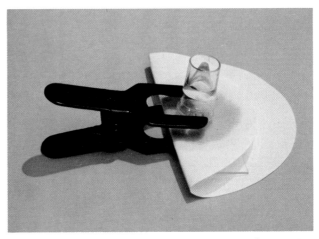

Fig 95. Preparation of the smear using the sedimentation method.

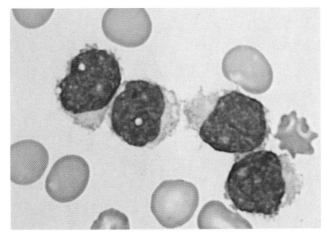

Fig 93. Artifact holes in the nuclei of mononuclear cells in the CSF.

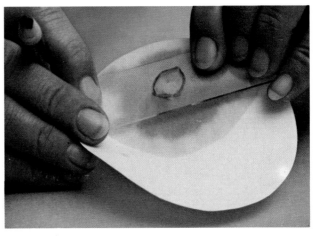

Fig 96. The finished specimen, using the sedimentation method, prior to staining of the smear.

Calcium pyrophosphate crystals measure 1–20 μ in length and up to 4 μ in width. They may be rectangles, rhomboids, or occasionally needles. The calcium pyrophosphate crystals show much weaker birefringence than the uric acid crystals.

When crystals have been identified with polarized light, the separation of urate from calcium pyrophosphate crystals can be made by using a first-order red compensator. The compensator retards red light so the field background is red instead of black. The orientation of the crystals to the axis of the compensator determines their birefringent properties. The long axis of the crystal is lined up parallel to the axis of slow vibration of the compensator (parallel to the compensator) by rotating the stage of the microscope. If the crystal is blue in this position, the crystal is calcium pyrophosphate and is positively birefringent. If it is yellow in this position, one is dealing with uric acid crystals, which are negatively birefringent with a compensator in place. When the stage is rotated 90° so that the long axis is perpendicular to the axis of the slow vibration of the compensator, the uric acid crystal turns from yellow to blue, while calcium pyrophosphate turns from blue to yellow (Fig 97).

It must be recognized, however, that optical designs of microscopes vary considerably from manufacturer to manufacturer. Therefore, the color that crystals assume in a particular direction may differ, depending on the type of microscope used. It is important to follow the manufacturer's directions and to use control slides. Also, with multi-headed microscopes, the direction or position of the image may vary from one microscope head to another.

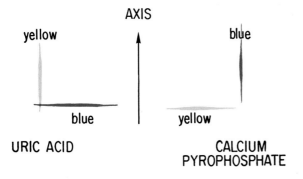

Fig 97. Two-dimensional representation of uric acid and calcium pyrophosphate crystals under polarized light using a red compensator.

In summary, the uric acid crystals are needle-shaped, strongly birefringent with a straight polarized light, and show a yellow, negative sign of birefringence when examined with a first-order red compensator. Calcium pyrophosphate crystals may be rod-shaped, needle-shaped, or appear as plates. They are weakly birefringent with polarized light and give a blue, positive sign of birefringence with a red compensator.

Under polarized light, corticosteroids may have an identical appearance to uric acid or calcium pyrophosphate crystals. Therefore, it is essential to know whether a previous intra-articular injection was given. Such crystals may be present in synovial fluid for a month or longer following the injection.

Cholesterol crystals appear as strongly birefringent plates, often with notched margins. Occasionally, they may have the appearance of needles or rhomboids similar to uric acid and calcium pyrophosphate crystals.

Fragments of cartilage may also be birefringent under polarized light but have irregular margins in contrast to the distinct, smooth parallel margins of uric acid or calcium pyrophosphate crystals. Other birefringent materials include dirt with unclean glassware and talcum crystals. The latter have a Maltese-cross appearance.

Comments

When multiple crystals are present, as may be seen when a tophus has been aspirated, it is easy to identify the type of crystal present. Frequently, however, the number of crystals is small, and several slides have to be carefully examined. It is recommended that a good polarizing microscope with a rotating stage be available. A satisfactory system can be devised by purchasing a polarizer set that includes a red compensator, and adding that to a standard laboratory microscope.

A control or reference slide is extremely useful. A reference slide can be made from a smear of uric acid crystal aspirated from a tophus. Such a reference slide will last for several years. A suspension of betamethasone acetate corticosteroid, which has a similar appearance to uric acid crystals under compensated polarized light, may also be used as a control slide.[9] The control slides should be rimmed with nail polish or a similar sealing material.

References

1. Tang TT, McCreadie SR: A simplified method for the cytologic study of body fluids. Am J Clin Pathol 59:113–116, 1973
2. Chu JY, Freiling P, Wassilak S: Simple method for the cytologic examination of cerebrospinal fluid. J Clin Pathol 30:486–487, 1977
3. Nishimura K, Hosoya R, Nakajima K: Sedimentation cytology in central nervous system leukaemia with a new simple apparatus. Br J Haematol 40:583–586, 1978
4. Kolmel HW: Atlas of Cerebrospinal Fluid Cells, ed 2. New York: Springer-Verlag, 1977
5. Oehmichen M: Cerebrospinal Fluid Cytology. An Introduction and Atlas. Philadelphia: WB Saunders Co, 1976
6. Hoeltge GA, Furlan A, Hoffman GC: The differential cytology of cerebrospinal fluids prepared by cytocentrifugation. Cleve Clin Q 43:237–246, 1976
7. Evans DIK, O'Rourk C, Jones PM: The cerebrospinal fluid in acute leukemia of childhood: Studies with the cytocentrifuge. J Clin Pathol 27:226–230, 1974
8. Choi HH, Anderson PJ: Diagnostic cytology of cerebrospinal fluid by the cytocentrifuge method. Am J Clin Pathol 72:931–943, 1979
9. Krieg AF: Cerebrospinal fluid and other body fluids, in Henry JB (ed): Clinical Diagnosis and Management by Laboratory Methods, ed 16. Philadelphia: WB Saunders Co, 1979, pp 635–679

Index